On the nature of human plasticity

On the nature of human plasticity

RICHARD M. LERNER

The Pennsylvania State University

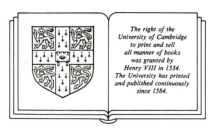

The right of the
University of Cambridge
to print and sell
all manner of books
was granted by
Henry VIII in 1534.
The University has printed
and published continuously
since 1584.

CAMBRIDGE UNIVERSITY PRESS

Cambridge
London   New York   New Rochelle
Melbourne   Sydney

Published by the Press Syndicate of the University of Cambridge
The Pitt Building, Trumpington Street, Cambridge CB2 1RP
32 East 57th Street, New York, NY 10022, USA
296 Beaconsfield Parade, Middle Park, Melbourne 3206, Australia

First published 1984

Printed in the United States of America

Library of Congress Cataloging in Publication Data
Lerner, Richard M.
On the nature of human plasticity.
Includes bibliographical references and index.
1. Adaptability (Psychology)   2. Adaptation (Biology)
3. Adaptability (Psychology) – Social aspects.   I. Title.
BF335.L47   1984   155   83-26138
ISBN 0 521 25651 8

TO ORVILLE G. BRIM, JR., AND JEROME KAGAN

Exemplary scholars and scientists,
Valued colleagues and friends

Contents

Foreword

Plasticity is a concept whose significance in developmental scholarship waxes and wanes, as the past decades of this century bear witness. For example, the term was a major entry in the 1902 edition of J. M. Baldwin and E. P. Poulton's *Dictionary of Philosophy and Psychology*. It was defined as "that property of living substance or of an organism whereby it alters its form under changed conditions of life" (Vol. 2, p. 302). At that time and under the recent influence of Darwinian thought, the discussion of plasticity focused on its origins and role in evolution. In the thirties and forties, plasticity (or modifiability) was again a center of attention. There was Lashley's conception of brain plasticity as well as the early-childhood studies of the detrimental impact of environmental deprivation and, correspondingly, the possible benefits of compensatory programs.

The 1970s and 1980s have seen renewed interest in the notion of plasticity. Research, rather than being restricted to childhood, is now being done, for example, in psychological gerontology, where it has been found that aging is not a fixed general process of decline, but rather that the older organism retains considerable potential for variability and plasticity. Similarly, in continuation of Lashley's earlier ideas, groundbreaking work is now being done in developmental psychobiology (e.g., Gollin, 1981) that underscores the need to study and articulate models that explicitly focus on variations in development.

There are several ways to interpret this continuation and transformation of interest in the concept of plasticity. My favorite is to view these developments as the direct expression of some basic tensions inherent in the developmental enterprise.

On the one hand, the study of development is characterized by a search for universal processes and mechanisms of ontogenetic change. On the other hand, as soon as movement toward the establishment of highly regularized processes of development occurs, a counterforce emerges challenging the existence of such universality. This counterstream is fed by several wells. There is foremost the notion that, as soon as mechanisms for development are found and understood, there is also a growing insight into the conditions that control these mechanisms.

ix

Thus, knowledge about the course and mechanisms of development spells also knowledge about its alterations.

Another reason for the recurring interest in the concept of plasticity is that the field of behavioral development is also intrinsically a field of application. The study of development encompasses not only description and explanation, but also efforts at modification and optimization. Thus, the concept of development entails value judgments about what constitutes progress (Nisbet, 1980) and how such progress can be achieved. As a consequence, many developmentalists are committed to studying not only how development looks, where it comes from, and how it comes about, but also what it could be if conditions were different. In this vein, the never-ending search for the potential (plasticity) of the organism is a cornerstone of developmental scholarship. A corollary implication is that, were the range of plasticity to be fully understood, the major raison d'être for further research on the nature of development would be in jeopardy.

In the present book, Lerner excels in articulating the current issues in research on plasticity in human development. But he also succeeds in moving the state of the art (see also Brim & Kagan, 1980) toward a new level of precision and of integration. I am particularly impressed with Lerner's abilities in three respects: first, his methodological and theoretical acumen in approaching plasticity as a multilevel and relativistic phenomenon. This permits him, for instance, to make explicit that we are moving beyond a dichotomous and absolutist view of the constancy versus change issue. The malleable and the unmalleable travel together. They are bonded to each other not like the opposite sides of the same coin, but like forces that give shape to each other. Second, Lerner's substantive reach – as evinced, for example, in his coverage of all periods of the life span from conception to death – sets new standards for a single-authored volume in the field. Similarly, Lerner adduces concepts and data from a wide range of disciplines, a feat rarely accomplished in this era of specialization.

Despite my positive regard, I am convinced that Lerner's book will be criticized because of his commitment to interdisciplinary breadth, willingness to speculate, and penchant for exploring the unknown. Anyone who is settled comfortably in his or her territory may not want to travel the road of cross-disciplinary dialogue and nonmainstream scholarship and may find fault in Lerner's work. I am persuaded that those who join the traveling party will enjoy, among other benefits, the pleasure of viewing some promising new terrain.

Paul B. Baltes
Berlin (FRG)

Preface

Over the course of the last decade or so exciting changes have occurred in those areas of social science that focus on human development. A growing number of studies of infants and children, of adolescents, and of adults and the elderly have yielded results challenging long-held views about the nature of human development: that early experience virtually immutably shapes the entire life course; that development is essentially a within-the-person phenomenon, largely unaffected in quality or quantity by the context of life; and that, by and large, all people develop in fairly standard, normative ways.

The recent studies indicate that people are more resilient to early, often quite negative experiences than was previously thought, that the events of early life do not necessarily constrain developments later on. They also suggest that features of the person's historical setting may sometimes shape personality and social and intellectual functioning much more than maturational- or age-associated changes. General events such as wars, economic privations, and political upheavals, as well as personal events such as marriage, divorce, illness, death, and career change, often profoundly affect both the quantity of life changes and the quality of the life course. Recent studies also indicate that there are multiple paths through life. As people age they become increasingly different from each other and, again, these different life paths are linked to general historical or personal life events. Finally, the active role of the person, in promoting both changes in self and context, has been indentified. By influencing their own development directly, and indirectly – by changing the context that feeds back to influence them – people are seen as producers of their own development.

These findings pressed many studying human development toward a new life-span perspective. Those taking this perspective emphasize that the potential for change exists across life, that as a consequence of the reciprocal interaction of active people in a changing world the life course is always characterized by the potential for *plasticity*, that is, systematic changes within the person in his or her structure and/or function. While not denying that constancies and continuities can, and do, characterize much of many people's life courses, and that plasticity is therefore not limitless, those taking the life-span perspective hold that many constancies and continuities are not necessary ones. They contend that change and the potential for change characterize life because of the plasticity of the processes involved in people's lives. From the level of biology to that of culture, these processes are presumed to be open to change – on the basis of both their inherent character (e.g., could a life process be adaptive if it were not capable of change?) and their reciprocal relations (their embeddedness) with other processes.

The existence of plasticity is not a point of minor practical significance. If all levels of life are open to change, then there is great reason to be optimistic about the ability of intervention programs to enhance human development.

To what extent are these life-span perspective views of change and plasticity tenable? In 1980, Orville G. Brim, Jr., and Jerome Kagan edited a volume (*Constancy and Change in Human Development*) that reviewed evidence from several disciplines pertinent to these views. The weight of the evidence lent support to these life-span conceptions. The present volume attempts to build on this earlier, significant effort. My goal is to extend the analyses found in Brim and Kagan's volume by reviewing current evidence for the existence of plasticity. I will discuss evidence from levels of analysis ranging from the genetic through the neuroanatomical, neurochemical, evolutionary biological, comparative–developmental, to the sociocultural within a common conceptual framework, one that encompasses descriptions of plasticity at each level as contributing to plasticity at all others. By emphasizing the idea of reciprocal interactions – each level of analysis being influenced by and influencing all others – I hope to build a rationale for the need for multidisciplinary research and intervention. Moreover, I hope to argue that to the extent that there is plasticity, it is appropriate to be optimistic about the ability of multidisciplinary research and intervention efforts to enhance human life.

I owe several debts of gratitude for the existence of this book. I completed my literature review for this book in November 1982. However, much of the work on this book was done while I was a 1980–81 Fellow at the Center for Advanced Study in the Behavioral Sciences. I am grateful for financial support provided by National Institute of Mental Health Grant #5-T32-MH14581-05 and by the John D. and Catherine T. MacArthur Foundation, and for the assistance of the Center's staff. Many of my co-Fellows provided stimulation and generous amounts of their time in order to facilitate my work on this book: Herbert Adams, Arthur S. Goldberger, Philip C. Kendall, Louis Lasagna, Gardner Lindzey, Dale T. Miller, and most especially Ruth T. (Toby) Gross. It was Toby Gross who first prompted me to read and think about many of the topics represented in this book.

In fact, if it were not for her stimulation, guidance, wisdom, and friendship, this book would not be a reality. I will always be greatly appreciative.

Since leaving the Center and through this writing my research and scholarly activities have been supported in part by a grant from the John D. and Catherine T. MacArthur Foundation. I am greatly appreciative to the Foundation for their support.

I am also grateful to the Foundation for Child Development for a consultantship that I held during the 1980–81 academic year, which gave me the opportunity to devote myself to the issues I treat in this book. I am also grateful to the Aspen Institute for Humanistic Studies for permitting me to organize and co-chair, with Orville G. Brim, Jr., a conference, supported by the Foundation for Child Development, on Enhancing Human Development and Change in the First Twenty Years of Life; at that conference an early draft of this book was presented. The feedback and direction I received from my fellow conference participants – Orville G. Brim, Jr., Jeanne Brooks-Gunn, Joel Charrow, W. Edward Craighead, Patricia H. Ellison, Jessie K. Emmet, Frank Furstenberg, Jr., Jerome Kagan, James G. Kelly, Miriam Kelty, Philip C. Kendall, Martha McClintock, Ross D. Parke, Anne C. Petersen, Victor Rouse, and Roberta Simmons – proved invaluable.

The feedback and criticism of several colleagues at Penn State and elsewhere have also been of great help to me. I thank Paul B. Baltes, Jay Belsky, Jack Block, J. Merrill Carlsmith, Roger A. Dixon, David L. Featherman, William T. Greenough, Christopher K. Hertzog, David F. Hultsch, Jacqueline V. Lerner, Kevin Mac Donald, David Magnusson, John W. Meyer, Walter Mischel, John R. Nesselroade, David S. Palermo, Matilda W. Riley, L. Alan Sroufe, James R. Stellar, Alexander von Eye, Mary Jo Ward, and Joachim F. Wohlwill.

Ross D. Parke and Orville G. (Bert) Brim deserve special mention. Ross Parke read several drafts of the manuscript and each time generously gave me the benefit of his broad and deep scholarship and insight. His contributions proved invaluable to me, and I am greatly appreciative. Bert Brim was a source of continuing intellectual stimulation and unwavering personal support. Writing a book is never an easy task. However, having Bert Brim to discuss my ideas with, to critique my work, and to bolster my spirit when the task seemed too difficult, was an invaluable experience for which I am deeply grateful.

I am especially thankful to Kathie Hooven, who typed the entire manuscript. Her patience and professionalism are truly remarkable. I also wish to thank several of my graduate students – Athena Droogas, Patricia L. East, Nancy Galambos, Karen Hooker, Marjorie B. Kauffman, M. Bernadette Riedy, and Michael Windle – who provided needed stimulation and important criticism. Patricia L. East and Marjorie B. Kauffman also assisted me in several of the clerical tasks necessary to complete the manuscript, and I thank them for their efforts.

I owe my greatest intellectual debt to Orville G. Brim, Jr., and Jerome Kagan – to whom this book is dedicated. Their scholarly and scientific efforts in exploring the issues I attempt to address in this book represent standards for all who follow.

Finally, and not at all least important, I thank my wife Jacqueline Lerner, my son Justin Samuel, and my daughter Blair Elizabeth, for bearing with an all-too-often absent husband and father and for giving him the love and encouragement to finish this task.

Richard M. Lerner
University Park

1   Perspectives on plasticity

In recent years, many social scientists (e.g., Baltes, Reese, & Lipsitt, 1980; Clarke & Clarke, 1976; Brim & Kagan, 1980) have been seriously questioning long-held conceptions of human development stressing constancy or continuity across life (e.g., see Fraiberg, 1977; Klaus & Kennell, 1976). The alternative view that has been emerging, based on increasing research evidence at levels of analysis ranging from the genetic to the cultural, stresses instead human plasticity at multiple levels of being (e.g., Cotman & Nieto-Sampedro, 1982; Greenough & Green, 1981; McClearn, 1981). Indeed, both theoretical and empirical work increasingly support the conviction that processes at any one of these levels of analysis may be linked to processes at every other level (e.g., Brent, 1978a; Magnusson, 1981; Magnusson & Allen, 1983; Prigogine, 1978, 1980).

Such developments call for a multidisciplinary reappraisal of the nature and bases of plasticity in human functioning and development and hold out the promise that multilevel multidisciplinary research and intervention will further increase behavioral plasticity and enhance human development. This revised view of the science of human behavior, which stresses complex interrelationships among the levels of human functioning – the inner biological, individual psychological, group and social network, societal, cultural/historical, and so on (Bronfenbrenner, 1977, 1979; Sarbin, 1977) – offers a perspective on causality that differs from past conceptions (Overton & Reese, 1981) and once again underscores the need for scientists to attend to the role that personal values and beliefs play in their research and intervention efforts (cf. Toulmin, 1981).

Perhaps the best summary description of the components and implications of this emerging view of the science of studying human behavior has been given by Roger Sperry, corecipient of the 1981 Nobel Prize in Medicine. Sperry (1982a) indicated that among the more important results of his split-brain work on brain–behavior relations was the derivation of a revised concept of the nature of consciousness, of an understanding of its fundamental relation to brain processing, and of a fundamental revision of what science stands for. He explains:

1

The key development is a switch from prior noncausal, parallelist views to a new causal, or "interactionist" interpretation that ascribes to inner experience an integral causal control role in brain function and behavior. In effect, and without resorting to dualism, the mental forces of the conscious mind are restored to the brain of objective science from which they had long been excluded on materialist–behaviorist principles.

The spreading acceptance of the revised causal view and the reasoning involved carry important implications for science and for scientific views of man and nature. Cognitive introspective psychology and related cognitive science can no longer be ignored experimentally, or written off as "a science of epiphenomena" or as something that must in principle reduce eventually to neurophysiology. The events of inner experience, as emergent properties of brain processes, become themselves explanatory causal constructs in their own right, interacting at their own level with their own laws and dynamics.

The whole world of inner experience (the world of the humanities), long rejected by 20th-century scientific materialism, thus becomes recognized and included within the domain of science.

Basic revisions in concepts of causality are involved, in which the whole, besides being 'different from and greater than the sum of the parts,' also causally determines the fate of the parts, without interfering with the physical or chemical laws of the subentities at their own level. It follows that physical science no longer perceives the world to be reducible to quantum mechanics or to any other unifying ultra element or field force. The qualitative, holistic properties at all different levels become causally real in their own form and have to be included in the causal account. Quantum theory on these terms no longer replaces or subsumes classical mechanics but rather just supplements or complements.

The results add up to a fundamental change in what science has long stood for throughout the materialist–behaviorist era (Sperry, 1981). The former scope of science, its limitations, world perspectives, views of human nature, and its societal role as an intellectual, cultural, and moral force all undergo profound change. Where there used to be conflict and an irreconcilable chasm between the scientific and the traditional humanistic views of man and the world (Jones, 1965; Snow, 1959), we now perceive a continuum. A unifying new interpretative framework emerges (Sperry, 1982b) with far-reaching impact not only for science but for those ultimate value–belief guidelines by which mankind has tried to live and find meaning (Sperry, 1982a, p. 1226).

The concept of plasticity is central to the research and conceptual analysis associated with the perspective illustrated by Sperry (1965, 1982a, 1982b; see too Gollin, 1981; Huxley, 1958; Schneirla, 1957; Willis, 1982). This concept, however, has been defined in several ways (cf. Franklin & Doyle, 1982; Gollin, 1981; Sigman, 1982). For instance, Sigman (1982, p. 98) notes that "the concept of plasticity is central to all biological and psychological studies of development. The concept signifies that the living organism can be modified by the environment. Any time we measure development or behavior of a subject in response to a stimulus, we are measuring plasticity." In turn, Gollin (1981, p. 231) indicates that plasticity refers to "the possible range of variations that can occur in individual development" (Gollin, 1981, p. 231) or to systematic structural and/or functional changes in a process, and may involve "variations that lie on a continuum of variation around some hypothesized average value, and variations that entail structural and functional changes of a qualitative nature" (Gollin,

1981, p. 237). However, several qualifications need to be made in order to make such general conceptions of plasticity more specific and useful.

Comparative versus ontogenetic perspectives

A cogent expression of the conception of plasticity that will be elaborated in those succeeding chapters that deal with evolutionary and comparative psychological bases of humans' potential for change across life was provided by Maier and Schneirla (1935). Remarking on ontogenetic differences among species, Maier and Schneirla observed that among members of species that reach their ultimate level of behavioral organization relatively early in life, behavior tends to be relatively stereotyped – that is, relatively "sense-dominated" (Hebb, 1949). On the other hand, members of species that take longer to reach their final level of behavioral organization are relatively more flexible: They can moderate their behaviors – for example, either approaching or withdrawing from a given stimulus – as circumstances require.

Maier and Schneirla were able to characterize differences among species on the basis of different species' contrasting capacities to modify behavior to adjust to new contextual circumstances (cf. Franklin & Doyle, 1982) – a view that serves to highlight species members' relative *flexibility*, that is, *the capacity to modify one's behavior to adjust to or fit with the demands of a particular context.* They emphasize, however, that this capacity may only be shown by a species at its most advanced level of development.

Two features of Maier and Schneirla's conception are important to emphasize here. First, the level of plasticity prototypical of a given species is not preformed; for instance, there is not a gene "coded" for plasticity such that whatever level of plasticity a species is capable of will be present either congenitally, or inevitably with age progression, in a member of that species (cf. Wilson, 1975). Instead, organisms must develop their plasticity; plasticity is a developmental phenomenon.

Second, Maier and Schneirla stress – and this often goes either unrecognized or unemphasized – that they are describing only *relative* differences among species. For instance, among mammals, rats are more stereotyped and less plastic than are chimpanzees, which in turn are more stereotyped and less plastic than humans. Note, however, that these distinctions depict none of these species as either completely stereotyped or completely plastic. In regard to humans, then, although their final level of behavioral organization shows relatively greater plasticity (or better – as I will explain shortly – flexibility) than that of other species, this certainly does not mean that humans are totally plastic; it does not mean that there are no limits on the the organism's ability to change across life, or that some unmodifiability – or stereotypy, in Schneirla's (1957) terms – does not remain with the organism across life. Indeed, Maier and Schneirla would likely argue that both types of functional characteristics may, in different circumstances, be useful for the organism; for example, plasticity of response may be useful when the organism behaves in contexts with rapidly changing or ambiguous cues for adjustment, whereas response stereotypy may be useful in contexts requiring rapid and/or numerous reflex-like responses for adjustment.

Another point needs to be made concerning Maier and Schneirla's contention that plasticity in any species and (probably) at any point in the life span is a relative functional feature of an organism. From a perspective aimed at identifying development or change, the concept of plasticity is comprehensible only as a relativistic phenomenon – that is, only when considered in the context of features of the organism that are not plastic. In order to identify features of ontogeny that qualify to be labeled "development" and in order to measure change, one needs to posit some constancy; in order to identify development one needs to identify an invariant, to gauge change one needs to identify a constant (Baltes, Reese, & Nesselroade, 1977; Kaplan, 1983). Similarly, in order to identify and study the plasticity of an organism or a system one needs to identify constraints.

Indeed, constraints are imposed by the organismic features of the human, by his or her context, and by his or her experience (see Kendall, Lerner, & Craighead, in press). Nevertheless, humans are relatively more plastic than other species, and this greater degree of plasticity that differentiates humans from other species is the level that is normatively present in the human's "final," adult period of life. This suggests that humans possess a capacity for systematic change – that humans retain some flexibility – across much if not all of their adult years. Indeed, one goal of this book is to demonstrate that the degree to which such flexibility exists across the human life span is greater than many people previously believed.

At this point it should be noted that consideration of the two key elements of Maier and Schneirla's conception of plasticity – the developmental nature of plasticity and its relativistic (as opposed to absolute) character – raise further issues, discussed in the following sections.

Plasticity as process versus plasticity as product

The concept of "levels" has been a useful one in comparative analyses. The role of this concept in Maier and Schneirla's (1935) conception of plasticity has just been indicated. Other scientists (e.g., Anderson, 1972) and philosophers (e.g., Nagel, 1957) have also made use of the idea. For instance, one may analyze a behavior of an organism – for example, the movement of one of its limbs – through recourse to either a psychological/behavioral, physiological, or physical level of analysis. All approaches to the analysis are equally legitimate, and useful analysis at one level does not obviate the usefulness of analyses at the other levels (Sperry, 1982a).

Indeed, in studying the development of an organism, a key issue is how variables or processes having their primary loci at one level of analysis relate to those having their main loci at other levels (e.g., Harris, 1957; R. Lerner, 1976; Nagel, 1957; Schneirla, 1956, 1957). These levels may include the physiochemical, physiological, individual psychological, dyadic–familial–social network, physical–ecological, societal, cultural, and historical levels (e.g., see Anderson, 1972), and one can approach the developmental problem in either one or both of two ways: (1) One can take a unitemporal approach and assess how variables from different levels present at the same time combine to influence behavior; (2) one can take a multitemporal–multilevel approach and assess how cotemporal variables at one or more levels influence subsequent variables. In either case, one can approach the analytic task from a reductionistic and/or an interactionist perspective (Magnusson & Allen, 1983; Lerner, 1976; Nagel, 1957; Overton & Reese, 1973; Reese & Overton, 1970). For example, an approach to analyzing behavioral development exemplified by Schneirla (1957) entails (1) appraisal of both the unitemporal–multilevel and multitemporal–multilevel features of the problem; (2) demonstration of how each level can relate to another either unidirectionally or bidirectionally; and (3) demonstration of how the analysis involved in this problem involves phenomena both within the organism and in the organism's context. According to Schneirla:

> The critical problem of behavioral development should be stated as follows:
> 1) To study the organization of behavior in terms of its properties at each stage, from the time of egg formation and fertilization through individual life history; and
> 2) to work out the changing relationships of organic mechanisms underlying behavior;
> 3) always in terms of the contributions of earlier stages in the developmental sequence;
> 4) and in consideration of the properties of the prevailing developmental context at each stage. (Schneirla, 1957, p. 80)

Applying Schneirla's concept of levels to an analysis of the development of species or an individual's plasticity thus involves:

1. Studying how properties at each level of analysis contribute to or constrain, alone and in combination, plasticity in each period of life;
2. Assessing how processes at levels of analysis "lower" than the more molar behavioral one may remain constant or change in the means by which they contribute to or constrain plasticity in each successive period of life;
3. Determining how antecedent periods of life promote or constrain degrees of plasticity manifested at subsequent periods; and
4. Understanding how the context of the organism limits, induces (Gottlieb, 1976b), or permits the expression and/or further development of plasticity.

However, analysis is complicated by a limitation in our language. We need to distinguish between the developmental processes that contribute to the organism's plasticity and the outcome of those processes, which is plasticity of behavior. Indeed, there is no compelling reason to focus only on behavioral organization as our "dependent variable" or outcome – we can, for instance, consider neuronal organization as a dependent variable and genetic and neuro-chemical processes as an independent variable. We are thus faced with a situation wherein (1) any of the processes involved in the matrix of developmental co-variation influencing an organism can be considered an antecedent of some other level's plasticity *or* as an outcome of other levels' functioning; and therefore (2) the processes that contribute to an organism developing plasticity and to its final level of plasticity may themselves be considered plastic.

While a major goal of this book will be to provide evidence in support of the latter inference, saying that plastic processes result in plastic outcomes runs the risk of being unclear about whether we are speaking of antecedent processes or products of these processes. Moreover, speaking repeatedly of *plasticity* runs the additional risk of losing sight of the fact that we are speaking only of relative plasticity, that we seek to discover both those conditions that permit and those that constrain systematic change in the structure and/or function of other variables.

Plasticity and probabilistic epigenesis

To circumvent the potential dangers raised by linguistic limitations, I will suggest some conventions. First, we should keep clear that plasticity is a relative concept and that the issue for the study of behavioral development is – to summarize the above – to learn the unitemporal and multitemporal, and the organism and contextual, conditions that promote and/or constrain systematic change in struc-ture and/or function. The need to understand how processes that promote plas-ticity also promote constraints on change has similarly been emphasized by Gollin (1981), who also adopts a multilevel causal view of the bases of an organism's plasticity. More or less in agreement with Schneirla (1957), Gollin observes that the variables from these bases providing plasticity are due to the probabilistic character of their confluence (see too Gottlieb, 1970; Lerner, 1978). Gollin indicates that

the determination of the successive qualities of living systems, given the web of rela-tionships involved, is probabilistic. This is so because the number of factors operating conjointly in living systems is very great. Additionally, each factor and subsystem is capable of a greater or lesser degree of variability. Hence, the influence subsystems have upon each other, and upon the system as a whole, varies as a function of the varying states of the several concurrently operating subsystems. Thus, the very nature of living systems, both individual and collective, and of environments, assures the presumptive character of organic change.

Living systems are organized systems with internal coherence. The properties of the parts are essentially dependent on relations between the parts and the whole (Waddington,

1957). The quality of the organization provides opportunities for change as well as constraints upon the extent and direction of change. Thus, while the determination of change is probabilistic, it is not chaotic. (Gollin, 1981, p. 232)

Underscoring Gollin's idea of probabilistic development is Gottlieb's (1970) concept of *probabilistic epigenesis*, a term he uses "to designate the view that the behavioral development of individuals within a species does not follow an invariant or inevitable course, and, more specifically, that the sequence or outcome of individual behavioral development is probable (with respect to norms) rather than certain" (p. 123).

Gottlieb goes on to explain that

probabilistic epigenesis necessitates a bidirectional structure–function hypothesis. The conventional version of the structure–function hypothesis is unidirectional in the sense that structure is supposed to determine function in an essentially nonreciprocal relationship. The unidirectionality of the structure–function relationship is one of the main assumptions of predetermined epigenesis [cf. Lerner, 1976, 1980]. The bidirectional version of the structure–function relationship is a logical consequence of the view that the course and outcome of behavioral epigenesis is probabilistic: it entails the assumption of reciprocal efforts in the relationship between structure and function whereby function (exposure to stimulation and/or movement of musculoskeletal activity) can significantly modify the development of the peripheral and central structures that are involved in these events. (P. 123; bracketed references added)

Characterizing development as probabilistic-epigenetic directly implies that the processes involved in development are plastic ones. Scarr (1982) also links the ideas of probabilistic epigenesis and plasticity:

Two big questions have occupied developmental theorists from antiquity to the present day. . . . First, is the course of human development directed primarily by structures in the environment that are external to the person, or is development guided principally by the genetic program within? Second, is development primarily continuous or discontinuous? (P. 852)

Scarr's first question bears on the idea of probabilistic epigenesis, the second on the concept of plasticity. In regard to the first issue, Scarr (1982) explains that

answers to the first question have shifted in recent years from the. . .empiricist position to the. . .nativist view. Neonativist arguments, however, do not assume the extreme preformism of the early century. Development does not merely emerge from the precoded information in the genes. Rather, development is a *probabilistic* result of indeterminate combinations of genes and environments. Development is genetically guided but variable and probabilistic because influential events in the life of every person can be neither predicted nor explained by general laws. Development, in this view, is guided primarily by the genetic program through its multilevel transactions with environments that range from cellular to social. The genetic program for the human species has both its overwhelming commonalities and its individual variability because each of us is both human and uniquely human. (Pp. 852–3)

In regard to the second question, Scarr (1982) suggests that because behavior depends upon both an organism's biological processes and the (probabilistic) transactions of these processes with its multilevel context, neither complete consistency nor complete change can be said to characterize the human condition:

Human beings are made neither of glass that breaks in the slightest ill wind nor of steel that stands defiantly in the face of devastating hurricanes. Rather, in this view, humans are made of the newer plastics – they bend with environmental pressures, resume their shapes when the pressures are relieved, and are unlikely to be permanently misshapen by transient experiences. When bad environments are improved, people's adaptations improve. Human beings are resilient and responsive to the advantages their environments provide. Even adults are capable of improved adaptations through learning, although any individual's improvement depends on that person's responsiveness to learning opportunities. (P. 853)

Scarr thus concludes that "one can be optimistic about human development, as early maladaptations do not necessarily foretell lifelong problems" (p. 853).

Focusing on the developmental processes underlying human plasticity thus leads us to characterize development as probabilistic-epigenetic, in which the organism's biology and its context interrelate reciprocally (Gottlieb, 1970, 1976a, 1976b; Lerner, 1976, 1978, 1980). Furthermore, development, especially as depicted by Werner's (1948, 1957) orthogenetic principle, represents a synthesis both of processes that act to make us the same through life and of processes that serve to continually change us. As emphasized earlier, we need constancy to identify and study change and, conversely, constancy cannot be identified or verified unless there is some change – for example, as in needing two times of measurement to identify stability.

This formulation of a probabilistic-epigenetic view of the relation between constancy and change is not without precedent (cf. Brim & Kagan, 1980; Werner, 1957). Indeed, a comparable position was taken early in the century by Baldwin and Poulton (Baldwin, 1902; Baldwin and Poulton, 1902), who explicated a relationship between constancy and change, in respect to both phylogeny and ontogeny, in their discussion of the concept of plasticity. Defining plasticity as "that property of living substance or of an organism whereby it alters its form under changed conditions of life" (Baldwin & Poulton, 1902, p. 302), they went on to discuss issues pertinent to the origin and manifestation of plasticity. They indicate that

the two theories of the manifestation of plasticity hold respectively (1) that it is a response to stimulation from the environment, the original property being simply general instability of structure not involving tendencies towards specific modifications of any sort; and (2) that it takes the form of specific changes which are inherent in life as such, the environment playing a secondary and purely exciting role. This latter is the view of those who accept VITALISM.

As to the origin of plasticity, the views associated with the first theory mentioned above are (a) that it is merely the original instability of protoplasm, or (b) that it is due – especially in the higher forms, as is seen in the plasticity of the brain substance – to natural selection, and is a necessity for ontogenetic development. The second theory given above – that of vitalism – holds that plasticity of the specific sort which it accepts is a fundamental property of life and explains phylogenetic evolution. (Baldwin & Poulton, 1902, pp. 302–3)

Two points are of interest about the above statement. First, Baldwin and Poulton depict theories that may be differentiated on the basis of what today would be termed respectively a mechanistic or contextual–mechanistic position (Overton, in press) and an organismic, or more specifically a predetermined epigenetic–organismic position (Gottlieb, 1970; Lerner, 1980). Second, they suggest that both positions are concerned with the links among plasticity, ontogeny, and phylogeny, although in distinctly different ways. According to Gould (1977), whose work will be discussed in Chapter 6, the nature of the association between ontogeny and phylogeny (which has been an issue at least since Aristotle) may account for the evolutionary bases of human plasticity. However, what is noteworthy at this point in our discussion is that Baldwin and Poulton (1902), in attempting to reconcile the two theories of plasticity, offered a formulation that presaged both the evolutionary position of Gould (1977) and the probabilistic-epigenetic position of Schneirla (1957) and Gottlieb (1970, 1976a, 1976b). Baldwin and Poulton thus illustrate, in encapsulated form, a link I will try to draw in Chapters 6 and 7 between evolutionary biology and hominid evolution, on the one hand, and the probabilistic-epigenetic organismic view of ontogenetic development on the other; in other words, they argue for the sort of connection I will too try to defend among evolution, ontogeny, and human plasticity. Finally, they see a relationship between constancy and change compatible with the one presented in this chapter:

It is probable – or possible – that there are two forms of plasticity: (a) that of the living cell wherever found, and of the lowest organism, by which they respond to various sorts of stimulation; and (b) that of the differentiated and developed structures and organisms whose modifications and variations are within certain defined and well-marked limits for each. It is possible, indeed, that this latter case illustrates the natural selection of certain modifications, i.e., those which served useful ends. In this case the fixity of organic structure, together with its second plasticity, has been acquired by the gradual restriction of its original plasticity: thus, according to recent writers (Bailey, Williams, A. Sedgwick), heredity itself as a function may have arisen. *There would seem, however, to be no reason to doubt that both processes are true: (1) the gradual reduction of original plasticity and variability, securing certain organic structural results from which (2) as a basis, has arisen, through evolution, the relative plasticity of brain, nerve, &c., which allows newer, and especially intelligent, accommodations.*

Apart from vital plasticity in general, the facts of individual accommodation make the nature and limits of brain plasticity a matter of great interest. Plasticity underlies all acquisition – especially motor acquisition – and learning. As a matter of endowment, it is contrasted with the fixity of instinct and reflex action; a contrast which, on the psychological side, is seen as educability or the lack of it. (Baldwin & Poulton, 1902, p. 303; italics added)

In other words, to Baldwin and Poulton the evolution of organic matter into an organized system is a function that has countered the unconstrained and dispersive character of an unorganized or entropic system (cf. Brent, 1978b; Lerner & Busch-Rossnagel, 1981; Prigogine, 1978, 1980). Nevertheless, this evolution of organization has involved the emergence of a system (an organism) marked by *relative* plasticity of its structural and functional properties – a point we have seen emphasized by Maier and Schneirla (1935) and by Schneirla (1957) in their probabilistic-epigenetic view of development. From a decreasing organic plasticity evolved organismic plasticity; in other words, only within an organized and coherent system, Baldwin and Poulton contend, can plasticity emerge to counter fixity and provide the basis of adaptability, flexibility, and educability (cf. Brim & Kagan, 1980). Thus, as I have been emphasizing, only within a context – a system that constrains – can plasticity have meaning and functional significance.

Emphasizing probabilistic-epigenetic development implies that the processes that give humans their individuality and their plasticity are the same ones that provide for human commonality and constancies (cf. McClearn, 1981). Indeed, Jack Block (pers. comm., 1982) makes this point when he cautions that one should not use the term *plasticity* to imply that within the malleable system there is not a structure or structures. He notes that ''if individuals are self-initiating, self-organizing systems, responsive in dynamic ways to changing contexts, this is because they have within them various ego structures, cognitive structures, perceptual structures, [and] action or knowledge structures through which experience is apprehended [and] processed and behavior is forged.'' He states that the term *plasticity* does not ''have the implication of a self-organizing, self-initiating, resilient system.'' Block's points suggest adopting another convention in terminology, one that will allow us to distinguish between (1) probabilistic-epigenetic developmental processes that have plasticity as one key feature of their functioning and (2) the functioning of an organized (''structured'') system that derives from probabilistic-epigenetic development.

Plasticity and flexibility

Let us use the term *plasticity* to refer to the evolutionary and ontogenetic processes by which one develops one's capacity to modify one's behavior to adjust to, or fit, the demands of a particular context. These plastic processes may then be said to contribute to the development of what we will term *flexibility*. Thus, plastic developmental processes (both at a given moment and across time, and both within the organism and between it and its context) can produce behavioral organization that is flexible, that has the capability of changing appropriately to meet contextual requirements.

There is some precedent in the developmental literature for using the term *flexibility* in the sense suggested above. Jeanne and Jack Block (e.g., 1980) have defined a key dimension of behavioral organization as "ego resiliency," by which they mean flexibility of behavior control. For instance, an ego-resilient child can plan and delay his or her behavior under the appropriate circumstances and then, when contextual conditions change, show spontaneity, enthusiasm, and curiosity where appropriate. Thus, the ego-resilient child is marked by a flexible behavioral organization, one that effectively meets the demands of the context, that provides a "goodness of fit" (Lerner & Lerner, 1983; Thomas & Chess, 1977) with the pressures of the setting, and as such promotes adaptive interchange.

Similarly, Sroufe (1979), discussing the variables or processes that may be continuous in human personality, suggests that one need not conceive of continuity in terms of static personality traits. Instead, one may conceive of continuity in the quality of adaptation. For instance, effective early adaptation should relate to effective functioning in later life. More specifically, Sroufe (1979, pp. 834–5) observes that

one solution to the problem of continuity in individual development lies in seeking qualitative similarities in patterns of behavior over time, rather than behavioral identities. In this view, children play active roles in seeking solutions to a series of developmental issues. Assessments focus on how well the child is meeting developmental challenges, on the quality of the child's adaptation. It is at this level of abstraction that continuity can be demonstrated.

Indeed, to justify this level of abstraction Sroufe (1979) adopts a view compatible with the synthesis between continuity and discontinuity promoted by Werner (1948, 1957); additionally, Sroufe calls for the use of a conception that may be useful in depicting the processes involved in the organization of this synthesis, which is, in my own view, a conception such as probabilistic epigenesis. That is, Sroufe (1979, p. 835) believes that "behavior does change lawfully, but the person remains the same. Such an approach does not mean less emphasis on observable behavior but more emphasis on the meaning and organization of behavior and on affective constructs underlying that organization."

In sum, optimally what may be developed in development is the style or capacity: of adapting well to one's circumstances (Sroufe, 1979); of showing appropriate flexibility in response to changing contextual pressures (Block & Block, 1980); of attaining a good fit or congruence with one's context (Lerner & Lerner, 1983; Thomas & Chess, 1977); of having a behavioral repertoire marked by "ego resiliency" (Block & Block, 1980). Indeed, as Sroufe (1979, p. 835) has pointed out:

At the individual level, adaptation refers to children's active engagement of the environment, fitting and shaping themselves to that environment and effecting changes in the environment to satisfy needs. The child does not merely react to environmental events but seeks stimulation and selects and organizes behavior in terms of his or her own goals.

In other words, the development of flexibility is marked by the person's ability to influence the context that influences him or her, to act as a producer of his or her own development (Lerner, 1982; Lerner & Busch-Rossnagel, 1981): The development of flexibility is marked by the development of efficacy in self-regulation.

In essence, then, developmental processes are plastic in that they continually involve probabilistic-epigenetic transactions between organism and context. The outcome (ontogenetic product) of these developmental progressions consists of internal and behavioral structures affording human flexibility, the ability to change self and/or context to meet the demands of life, and the ability to attain a "good fit" with the context. (Cf. Chapter 9 for a discussion of a "goodness-of-fit" model of person–context relations, a model that is derived from a more general probabilistic-epigenetic person–social context model presented in Chapter 8 and that emphasizes the role of individuals as producers of their own development; Lerner, 1982; Lerner & Busch-Rossnagel, 1981.)

Plasticity as a relativistic conception

Much of the foregoing has indicated that plasticity is not limitless. Human behavior is always influenced by past events, current conditions, and the specific features of our organismic constitution. Indeed, I have argued above that a notion of complete or limitless plasticity is antithetical to any useful concept of development (Baltes, Dittmann-Kohli, & Dixon, 1982; Kaplan, 1983; Lerner & Busch-Rossnagel, 1981; Sroufe, 1979; Sroufe & Waters, 1977) and is therefore unwarranted on several grounds, including philosophical, theoretical, and methodological – as well as empirical (e.g., see Block, 1982). On the other hand, any view that stresses complete constraints, necessary connectivity across life periods, or irremedial limits placed on later behavioral organization by antecedent experiences would face similar philosophical, theoretical, and methodological problems – and would moreover be ignoring evidence for the existence of at least some behavioral flexibility across life (Baltes & Baltes, 1980; Baltes & Willis, 1982; Greenough & Green, 1981; Willis, 1982; Willis & Baltes, 1980) and of the plasticity of the processes producing such capability.

It deserves emphasizing here, however, that a critical analysis of the concept of plasticity – at least in terms of Schneirla's (1957) probabilistic epigenesis – does not boil down to determining whether it is constancy or change, whether it is stereotypy or plasticity, that characterizes development. All these do. Indeed, according to Werner's (1948, 1957) orthogenetic principle, a developmental change is *defined* as one wherein processes promoting discontinuity (i.e., those promoting differentiation) are synthesized with those promoting continuity (i.e., those promoting hierarchic integration). Developmental change, itself a synthesis of constancy and change, is thereby consistent with those features of ontogeny that are highlighted by a probabilistic-epigenetic conception of development.

Thus, the task for developmental analysis is one of determining the personal and contextual conditions under which one will see constancy or change (cf. Block, 1982; Lerner, 1979). For instance, what developmental processes lead to a child developing a given level of "ego resiliency" (Block & Block, 1980), and what conditions constrain the development of such a level of flexibility? To the extent that the processes enhancing or limiting such flexibility are plastic ones, we are prompted to raise a second question: Can the conditions constraining the development of flexibility – or continuing with our use of the Blocks' term, ego resiliency – be altered? A third question immediately arises: If we can alter these limits, should we? The next two sections of this chapter discuss the issues raised by the latter two questions.

The role of presuppositions in the study of development

If the processes leading to flexibility are plastic ones – that is, if variables at the multiple levels of analysis involved in development are themselves flexible and thus in combination constitute plastic developmental processes – then there is reason to believe that the products of these processes can be altered, specifically, that as our knowledge and technology increase, we may be able to enhance flexibility. Clearly, this is an optimistic inference, once admittedly associated with what may be labeled a "presupposition" of plasticity.

Kagan (1980, 1983) has discussed the role of "presuppositions" – culturally deep-rooted, preempirical ideas about the nature of reality – in the development of developmental psychology. Historically, many of the scientific disciplines devoted to the study of human behavior, its evolution and development, have been influenced by a "presupposition of limits" (Gould, 1981). This term, used here to embrace a general position or class of arguments in philosophy (see Toulmin, 1981), denotes the view that human functioning is unalterably constrained by a specified factor or set of factors (e.g., genes, early experience), that there is a necessary "connection" (cf. Kagan's, 1980, 1983, discussion of the presupposition of connectivity) between what arises from these causal variables and consequent forms or functions, and that this connection is inaccessible for manipulation or alteration (Lehrman, 1970). In other words, this view implies that there is one (or a limited few) developmental pathway(s), and that an individual's trajectory along a path is channeled by causal factors that permit no deviation.

Although most current conceptions of development that manifest this presupposition do not define it in as strong terms as outlined above, there are nevertheless relatively recent theoretical statements consistent with the presupposition of limits (e.g., Lorenz, 1965; Eysenck & Kamin, 1981). For instance, Klaus and Kennell's (1976) notion of mother–infant bonding stresses that the quality of the bond established in the first minutes or hours after birth imposes a potent constraint on the newborn's subsequent social and affective development. Klaus and Kennell (1976, pp. 65–6) state that they "strongly believe that an essential principle of attachment is that there is a *sensitive period* in the first minutes and hours after an infant's birth which is optimal for the parent-infant attachment," and go on to explain one of their principles of attachment: "Early events have long-lasting effects. Anxieties a mother has about her baby in the first few days after birth, even about a problem that is easily resolved, may affect her relationship with the child long afterward" (Klaus & Kennell, 1976, p. 52). Their conclusion is that

this original mother–infant bond is the wellspring for all the infant's subsequent attachments and is the formative relationship in the course of which the child develops a sense of himself. Throughout his lifetime the strength and character of this attachment will influence the quality of all future bonds to other individuals. (Klaus & Kennell, 1976, pp. 1–2)

Fraiberg (1977), assuming a conceptual position not dissimilar to Klaus and Kennell's, contends that throughout the life span, every expression of the emotion of love is necessarily connected to a bond that originated in the first year of life:

Love of a partner and sensual pleasure experienced with that partner begin in infancy, and progress to a culminating experience, "falling in love," the finding of a permanent partner, the achievement of sexual fulfillment. In every act of love in mature life, there is a prologue which originated in the first year of life. (Fraiberg, 1977, pp. 31–2)

Earlier developmental theories even more explicitly reflected the presupposition of limits. Broca's craniology in the nineteenth century posited that the size of the human skull is a factor limiting intellectual capacity (Gould, 1981). Similarly, genetic deterministic theories of both the previous and present centuries have assumed that individual biology – received at conception and represented by the genotype – constrains moral (Lorenz, 1940), cognitive (Goddard, 1912, 1914), or vocational (Terman, 1916) development (cf. Gould, 1981). In short, the presupposition of limits reflects a preempirical (and in my view unduly pessimistic) belief in the irremediable character of human nature: It holds that we are direct, unalterable products of our evolution, our biology, our genes; there can be no intervention to prevent, ameliorate, or enhance this "natural order."

In contrast, a presupposition of plasticity involves the belief that changes may take place over time in a person's physical, psychological, and social structures and functions. People always exist in a physical and social world that they both influence and are influenced by. Because of the reciprocal relations between people and their worlds one may be optimistic about the possibility of positive changes. The presupposition of plasticity underlies the hope that experiences at one time in life need not constrain possibilities later on, that at least some early problems, deficits, or insults to the integrity of the organism may be ameliorated (Scarr, 1982; Sigman, 1982).

Philosophical characteristics of the presuppositions. Toulmin (1981), observing that scientists often inadequately appreciate the ways in which their historical context and the concomitant, implicit philosophy they adopt constrain their understanding of their subject matter and of causality, uses the example of developmental psychology and specifically discusses the philosophical characteristics of the presuppositions of limits and of plasticity. He points out that just because a philosophical position is logically defensible – that is, legitimate in terms of internal coherence – is not a reason to accept its practical validity:

Any formal system, simply as such, possesses the kind of internal systematicity associated with logical necessity; yet no such formal system, simply as such, can guarantee its own pragmatic necessity, or indispensability. Many formal systems have initially been given an unrestricted practical application, only to have limits subsequently placed on them in the light of actual experience. (Toulmin, 1981, p. 260)

Toulmin, addressing the philosophical considerations surrounding the issue of the presupposition of limits versus that of plasticity, provides grounds for rejecting the concept of "universal destination" – that is, the concept of a single, generic life course having universal features:

To start with, all we need here is a "burden of proof" argument. What little evidence we have undercuts any supposition that intellectual evolution and conceptual development have a single, unique, and universal destination. At the very least, that evidence falls short of what we should need to raise this supposition to a basic axiom either of epistemology, or of developmental psychology. Whether as philosophers or as psychologists, it is therefore desirable that we should consider how the theoretical ambitions of both fields need to be reformulated, once the burden of proof is shifted: That is to say, if we take as our starting point the contrary supposition, that the directions of conceptual ontogeny and phylogeny alike are to some significant degree indeterminant and open-ended. (Toulmin, 1981, p. 257)

The arguments supporting this skepticism lead Toulmin (1981, p. 260) to contend that in all "spheres of thought and action...the claims for a unique, universal destination must be challenged...." Speaking of cognitive development, Toulmin challenges the view that there is a universal direction to development; more appropriate, he argues, is the position that many potential directions for development may exist:

What we have available for study in developmental psychology today is not the spectacle of young children "coming to recognize the necessity of" certain universal formal schemata: Rather, it is the processes by which they are in fact socialized and enculturated into the actual praxis, thought, and speech current in any culture sharing our particular kinds of technical sophistication. As to the question, how far, for example, animistic cultures share our façons de parler and façons de penser in considering substance and causality: That is an issue we must approach with open minds.... All cultures having any real degree of modernization and technical sophistication most probably share some substantial common elements: Whether in their ways of handling spatial relations, or material substance, or causality, or whatever. But the existence of substantial common elements is one thing: The supposition of a priori necessity is something quite else.* (Toulmin, 1981, p. 262)

In sum, Toulmin (1981) points out that all scientific endeavors are colored by philosophical beliefs and that one must remain open-minded to these. For our purposes, it is important to note that not only the logical viability but also the pragmatic advantage of adopting a presupposition of plasticity are grounds for optimism about human change.

Scientific and social policy implications of the presuppositions. Adopting the presupposition of plasticity implies adopting a scientific agenda – and social policy stance (Brim, 1982; Brim & Kagan, 1980) – that distinctly differs from that more readily promoted by adopting a presupposition of limits.

For example, the concepts of genetic inheritance and instinct as propounded by Konrad Lorenz (1940, 1965, 1966), it may be argued (Lehrman, 1953; Schneirla, 1956; Eisenberg, 1972), rely on a presupposition of limits. Lorenz (1940, 1965) argued that genetic inheritance represents a "blueprint" for development and behavior, a set of directives unalterable by environment, experience, learning, socialization, and so on (cf. Lehrman, 1953, 1970). Genetic inheritance, according to Lorenz, circumscribes behavior by leading directly to the formation of an "instinct," a preformed, innate, and unmodifiable pattern of species-specific behavior.

To understand Lorenz's use of this conception in regard to human behavior – and to appreciate how such a position can influence not just scientific activity but social policy as well – consider the following written by Lorenz (as translated by Eisenberg, 1972) in Nazi Germany in 1940:

The only resistance which mankind of healthy stock can offer... against being penetrated by symptoms of degeneracy is based on the existence of certain innate schemata.... Our

---

* Toulmin continues: "And the acknowledgement of substantial common elements, in some specific respects and to some recognizable extent, still leaves room for plenty of variety, both of kind and of degree.... The most that we are entitled to take for granted, surely, is that the practical demands of human life and experience in any particular sphere of thought and action will restrict the available destinations of mental development within a reasonably narrow compass. In this respect, the goal of philosophy from now on should no longer be to demonstrate the 'logical necessity' of any particular conceptual framework, or set of 'basic forms of thought.' Rather it should be to learn, from reflection on actual experience, how far and in what respects the 'pragmatic necessities' of our societal, cultural, and technical situations place constraints on the manual, intellectual, and other operations we employ in dealing with spatial relations, material commodities, and the rest: How far, and in what respects (on the contrary) they leave us with scope to choose, and to change, one set of basic operations and another." (pp. 262, 263–4).

species-specific sensitivity to the beauty and ugliness of members of our species is intimately connected with the symptoms of degeneration, caused by domestication, which threaten our race....Usually, a man of high value is disgusted with special intensity by slight symptoms of degeneracy in men of the other race...In certain instances, however, we find not only a lack of this selectivity...but even a reversal to being attracted by symptoms of degeneracy....Decadent art provides many examples of such a change of signs....The immensely high reproduction rate in the moral imbecile has long been established....This phenomenon leads everywhere...to the fact that socially inferior human material is enabled...to penetrate and finally to annihilate the healthy nation. The selection for toughness, heroism, social utility...must be accomplished by some human institution if mankind, in default of selective factors, is not to be ruined by domestication-induced degeneracy. *The racial idea as the basis of our state has already accomplished much in this respect.* The most effective race-preserving measure is...the greatest support of the natural defenses....We must – and should – rely on the healthy feelings of our Best and charge them with the selection which will determine the prosperity or the decay of our people. (Italics added)

Although switching his scientific focus from Jews to precocial birds after the Nazis lost the war, Lorenz maintained an interest in human instincts and continued to view them in a manner consistent with a presupposition of limits. In his book *On Aggression*, Lorenz (1966) argued that aggression is instinctual in humans, that social conflict is an innate component of the human behavioral repertoire, and that there is an instinctual "militant enthusiasm" among youth. Lorenz recommends that civilization find methods for ritualizing aggressive instincts as a means of containing them – that is, that we make the best of an inevitably negative situation (Schneirla, 1966), since humans are universally and unalterably destructively aggressive. The social policy implication of this instance of the presupposition of limits was perhaps best described in a review by Schneirla (1966, p. 16) of *On Aggression*:

It is as heavy a responsibility to inform man about aggressive tendencies assumed to be present on an inborn basis as it is to inform him about "original sin," which Lorenz admits in effect. A corollary risk is advising societies to base their programs of social training on attempts to inhibit hypothetical innate aggressions, instead of continuing positive measures for constructive behavior.

Conclusions. The issues raised by adopting a presupposition of plasticity as opposed to one of limits allow us to make three points. First, *all* scientific endeavors are based on philosophical assumptions or presuppositions (Kuhn, 1970; Overton & Reese, 1973; Pepper, 1942; Reese & Overton, 1970; Toulmin, 1981): Even the denial of this point is itself based on an implicit philosophical stance (Watson 1977). Second, these presuppositions provide more than contrasting sets of values, ideologies, theologies, and so on. In addition, they are associated with often quite distinct theoretical and methodological approaches to studying human development (Overton & Reese, 1973; Reese & Overton, 1970; Werner, 1957). Third, when scientific theory and data provide a basis of social policy, these presuppositions can be associated with conditions helping or hindering large segments of humanity.

Beliefs, values, and interventions

As used in the human development literature, the term *intervention* means an action that alters the direction or quality of life. Interventions need not be planned or intended; indeed, if we accept the idea that all human activities are potentially interconnected, then a failure to act, to intervene, is itself an intervention. By not acting we alter the matrix of interactions impinging on a person; we create a context different from that which would be created if we had in fact acted. Failure to intervene changes the contextual bases of a person's development and may itself be a potent, albeit unintentional, type of intervention.

People actively involved in the task of intervening typically plan their actions, often developing complex strategies and programs to alter health, behavior, nutrition, cognition, achievement, etc. To the extent that intervenors believe that human behavior, biology, morality, and so on cannot be altered, they will not act to intervene – although this nonaction is also an intervention. Thus, if presuppositions about the changeability of human functioning are wrong, inaction constitutes an intervention delimiting or constraining the promotion of those conditions potentially productive of change. One's inactions will create a self-fulfilling prophecy.

In short, the concept of fixity in human functioning and development suggests that humans are resistent to change, that they are static, immutable organisms, whereas the concept of plasticity suggests that there is some potential for within-person (intraindividual) change and that there is thus a point to studying processes fostering or constraining change.

Thus if we assume the existence of plasticity, we are led to an optimistic orientation to intervention. In addition to preventative strategies, techniques aimed at ameliorating or even enhancing the human condition may be appropriately instituted (Clarke & Clarke, 1976). Without such an assumption, people who possess undesirable characteristics are simply considered beyond remediation (Hunt, 1961). Similarly, if it is believed that one's genes or early life experiences have an unmodifiable connection to functioning at later life (Kagan, 1980; 1983), then rather severe treatment policies will be instituted to deal with "undesirables." In this connection Brim and Kagan (1980, p. 21) note that

the belief that early experiences create lasting characteristics, like the belief in biological and genetic determinism, makes it possible to assume that attempts to improve the course of human development after early childhood are wasted and without consequence. If society believes that it is all over by the third year of life, it can deal harshly with many people in later life because nothing more can be done, and social programs designed to educate, redirect, reverse, or eliminate unwanted human characteristics cannot be justified. Policies of racial, ethnic, and sex discrimination, incarceration rather than rehabilitation of criminals, ignoring urban and rural poverty, and isolation of the elderly have found shelter in the belief in the determinism of the early years of life.

In addition to Lorenz (1940, 1965, 1966), many others have held the view that genetically fixed or early developed limits and continuity characterize much of the human life course (see too Chess & Thomas, 1982; Gould, 1981). This view has variously been built on: (1) the premise of "connectivity" (Kagan, 1980; 1983), that the pattern of psychological life is irrevocably fixed by experiences in infancy and early childhood; (2) the idea that genetic inheritance provides an unalterable "blueprint" for the development of such psychological functions as intelligence (Hunt, 1961) or personality (e.g., Sheldon, 1940, 1942); and (3) the idea that psychological development follows species-specific instinctual functions (e.g., A. Freud, 1969) and that life after a certain point (usually adolescence) is characterized by stability or decline (Baltes et al., 1980). Each of these presuppositions leads directly to the position that changing human development from its normative channels is not feasible, especially after childhood or early adolescence.

In turn, the presupposition of plasticity leads in other conceptual and research directions. As noted earlier in this section, however, an important question regarding plasticity involves not beliefs and intervention but, instead, values and intervention: Even if we presuppose plasticity and believe that constraints on the actualization of human flexibility can be altered, *should* this be done? For example, with the virtual explosion in recent years in knowledge and technology in genetic engineering through recombinant DNA methodology (discussed in Chapter 3), scientists and society are faced with dilemmas such as "Should we create new forms of life?" and "Under what conditions may we ethically begin gene therapy in humans?" (e.g., see Anderson, 1982; Anderson & Fletcher, 1980; Hubbard, 1982; Walters, 1982).

Such decisions are complicated by the character of human plasticity itself. If behavioral flexibility results from plastic processes involving both the organism and its context, then promotion of greater flexibility at the level of the organism may be associated with undesired changes at other levels or at a later time (cf. Sigman, 1982). For example, promoting flexibility sufficient to allow a woman to successfully meet the demands simultaneously of the home (e.g., in regard to marriage and parental roles) and of the workplace (e.g., in regard to professional development) may be a change valued by the woman and by an intervenor; and such changes may be accompanied by other valued ones in the woman (e.g., her self-esteem and her personal income may be increased). However, unanticipated and undesired changes may ensue (cf. Block, 1973). For example, the woman's parents may disapprove of her working outside the home, and conflict may result.

Thus, plasticity is a "double-edged" sword: The promise of potential enhancement of the human condition is qualified by the potential of undesirable consequences of a change at the same or another level and even the possibility that the organism may be changed not for the better, but for the worse. Recognition of this ambiguous character of plasticity itself represents a limit on plasticity, for without some way of anticipating all the possible effects of intervention, we cannot accurately appraise the cost/benefit ratio of attempts to foster plastic developmental progressions. Although increased flexibility can be expected to permit a person greater leeway in adjusting to his or her context, not all changes that lead to or accompany such an increase will be necessarily adaptive for or valued by the person. Scientists and other interventionists are thus in a difficult ethical position regarding how to proceed with their work; in my view, only scientifically conservative steps are warranted (cf. Anderson & Fletcher, 1980).

The plan of this book

Succeeding chapters discuss the evidence for the presence of plastic processes at the several levels of analysis that comprise the subject matter of human development, demonstrate how plasticity at each level both derives from and contributes to plasticity at other levels, and argue that, given such plasticity, the potential exists for successful research and intervention aimed at actualizing the flexibility that may arise therefrom. The next chapter discusses the theoretical and empirical bases of an emerging perspective about the nature of the human condition, the *life-span view of human development*, which rests on the idea that as a consequence of reciprocal relations between individual and contextual processes the potential for change exists across life. Also, two key components of this perspective – what I label *embeddedness* and *dynamic interaction* – will be defined and elaborated to support the idea that individual development at multiple levels of analysis is a plastic phenomenon.

The major evidence for the presence of plasticity, and its import for multilevel research and intervention, has been derived from theory and research reviewed in Chapters 3 through 8, which focus on genetics, neuroanatomy, neurochemistry, evolutionary biology, anthropology, comparative developmental psychology, and sociology. Chapter 9 then discusses how the life-span perspective may be useful in extending multidisciplinary research and intervention efforts, and Chapter 10 presents my general conclusions.

Throughout these discussions I will cast my comments to address three questions:

1. Is there plasticity at multiple levels of analysis – for example, at the genetic, neuronal, and societal levels?

2. Does this plasticity both result from and enable reciprocal relations among levels of analysis?
3. Does this reciprocity provide a useful basis for multidisciplinary research and intervention?

By answering these questions in the affirmative, I hope to demonstrate that the presence of human plasticity warrants optimism regarding the ability of multi-disciplinary research and intervention to enhance human development and change.

2 The life-span view of human development: philosophical, historical, and substantive bases

Human development, or more accurately child development, was often studied in the first several decades of this century within university institutes – for example, at Iowa, Minnesota, and Berkeley. Although these centers originally took a multidisciplinary approach, the pluralistic perspective began to erode by the 1950s and was eventually replaced by a single view of development, the psychological (L. P. Lipsitt, pers. comm., December 1979; D. S. Palermo, pers. comm., August 1980; see also Hartup, 1978). The 1970s were marked by calls for a return to interdisciplinary integration (e.g., Brim & Kagan, 1980; Bronfenbrenner, 1977; Burgess & Huston, 1979; Hill & Mattessich, 1979; Lerner & Spanier, 1978; Petrinovich, 1979; Riley, 1979; Sarbin, 1977), calls motivated primarily by instances of failure to confirm some key hypotheses of developmental psychological analysis.

A case in point involves attempts to use a biological model of growth, one based on an idealized maturational (organismic) conception of development, to account for data from the adult and aged years (Baltes, et al., 1980; Baltes & Schaie, 1973). According to this type of organismic conception, the adult and aged years are periods of decline. However, much of the data regarding age changes (e.g., in intellectual performance) during these life periods turned out to be inconsistent with this paradigm. For example, pertinent data sets revealed increasingly greater differences in individual change: As people grow older, the differences between them apparently increase (Baltes, 1979a; Baltes & Schaie, 1974, 1976; Schaie, Labouvie, & Buech, 1973).

Regarding such data Brim and Kagan (1980, p. 13) conclude that ''growth is more individualistic than was thought, and it is difficult to find general patterns.'' More importantly, variables associated with when people are born (i.e., with membership in particular birth cohorts) and with other historical events appeared to account for more of these changes, particularly with respect to adult intellectual development, than did age-associated influences (Baltes et al., 1980). Data sets pertinent to children (Baltes, Baltes, & Reinert, 1970) and adolescents (Nesselroade & Baltes, 1974) also supported the saliency of these birth cohort and

22

time-of-measurement effects in developmental change. These findings induced scientists to develop conceptualizations useful for understanding the role of these non-age-related variables in development (e.g., Baltes, Cornelius, & Nesselroade, 1977; Brim & Ryff, 1980).

As a consequence of these theoretical and empirical developments, not only in developmental psychology but in life-course sociology as well (e.g., Brim, 1966, 1968; Riley, 1979), many social scientists altered the focus of their work, which consequently underwent a major conceptual change. Instead of dealing exclusively with ideas derived only from mechanistic or organismic paradigms, many began including a concern with contextually derived and contextually sensitive conceptions (see Baltes, 1979b; Bandura, 1982; Jenkins, 1974 Mischel, 1977; Sarbin, 1977). As explained by Overton (in press), this alteration often involved an attempt to combine ideas from organicism (e.g., pertaining to the organized and active nature of the organism) with those of another paradigm, that is, contextualism (Pepper, 1942); here the key ideas were those of the active context, of the role of normative and nonnormative events at multiple contextual levels (for instance, the family, the community, the society), and of the reciprocal relations between context and organism. This organismic–contextual focus promoted the evolution of a new perspective about human development. Brim and Kagan (1980, p. 1) have summarized the status of this alteration in orientation by noting that this conception of human development

differs from most Western contemporary thought on the subject. The view that emerges. . . is that humans have a capacity for change across the entire life span. It questions the traditional idea that the experiences of the early years, which have a demonstrated contemporaneous effect, necessarily constrain the characteristics of adolescence and adulthood. . . . there are important growth changes across the life span from birth to death, many individuals retain a great capacity for change, and the consequences of the events of early childhood are continually transformed by later experiences, making the course of human development more open than many have believed.

The perspective characterized by Brim and Kagan (1980) has led to a renewed concern with issues of relations between evolution and ontogeny (Baldwin & Poulton, 1902; Maier & Schneirla, 1935; Schneirla, 1957; Tobach, 1978; Tobach & Schneirla, 1968), of constancy and change (Brim & Kagan, 1980; Lerner, 1976; Werner, 1957), of human plasticity (Gollin, 1981; Schneirla, 1957; Sigman, 1982), and of the role people play in their own development (Lerner, 1982; Lerner & Busch-Rossnagel, 1981; Sroufe, 1979). As I will discuss in more detail below, these issues are linked by the idea that reciprocally deterministic (i.e., dynamic) interactions (Lerner, 1978, 1979) between individuals and their multiple contexts characterize human development. For example, from this perspective biological variables both influence and are influenced by behavioral and social ones (Petersen & Taylor, 1980; Sperry, 1982a); as a consequence of this social embeddedness, biological and behavioral processes are seen both as plastic in character and as assuring plasticity. All the issues raised by this emerging perspective derive from a common appreciation of the basic role of the changing context in developmental change. This appreciation is reflected in the growing commitment among many social scientists to expand their disciplinary expertise by gaining an understanding of the relations among levels of analysis with the aim of creating a broadened multidisciplinary knowledge base.

General propositions of the life-span perspective

The consequence of all this empirical and conceptual activity has been the crystallization of the perspective labeled *life-span developmental psychology* or the *life-span view of human development* (Baltes, 1979a; Baltes, et al., 1980). The nature of this orientation has emerged over the course of several conferences (Baltes & Schaie, 1973; Datan & Ginsberg, 1975; Datan & Reese, 1977; Goulet & Baltes, 1970; Nesselroade & Reese, 1973), the initiation of publication of an annual volume devoted to life-span development (Baltes, 1978; Baltes & Brim, 1979, 1980, 1981), and the publication of numerous empirical and theoretical papers (Baltes, 1979b; Baltes & Nesselroade, 1973; Baltes, et al., 1980; Featherman, 1981–2). From this scholarly activity, it has become clear that one may thus characterize the life-span perspective as a set of interrelated ideas about the nature of human development and change. In combination these ideas present a set of implications for theory building, for methodology, and for scientific collaboration across disciplinary boundaries.

Two key propositions or assumptions of the life-span perspective may be labeled *embeddedness* (Lerner, Skinner, & Sorell, 1980) and *dynamic interaction* (Lerner, 1978, 1979, in press). From these propositions may be derived an interrelated set of implications; together, these propositions and implications constitute the key concepts in current life-span thinking.

Embeddedness and dynamic interactionism

The idea of embeddedness is that the key phenomena of human life exist at multiple levels of being (inner biological, individual psychological, dyadic, social network, community, societal, cultural, outer physical–ecological, historical, etc.); at any one point in time variables and processes from any and all of these multiple levels may contribute to human functioning. Moreover, these levels do not function in parallel, as independent domains; rather, variables and processes at all levels are reciprocally influential: There is a dynamic interaction among levels. This idea is, as noted in Chapter 1, a key component of the probabilistic-epigenetic view of development (Gottlieb, 1970, 1976a, 1976b; Lerner, 1978, 1980; Scarr, 1982).

Moreover, as I will now discuss, the assumptions of embeddedness and dynamic interaction found in the life-span perspective are associated not only with an organismic view of development, but importantly, also are associated with what may be labeled a "contextual" (Pepper, 1942) paradigm of development (cf. Overton, in press). It is of use to discuss the features of this paradigm, and indicate how it relates to the key propositions of a life-span perspective and to a probabilistic-epigenetic conceptualization of development.

Features of a contextual view of development. Knowledge about psychological development has traditionally been advanced most notably by research derived from either an organismic or mechanistic paradigm (Baltes, 1979b; Overton & Reese, 1973; Reese & Overton, 1970). Although contributions derived from the two paradigms have remained relatively unintegrated (Kuhn, 1978; Overton, 1983), the paradigms nevertheless share certain assumptions (cf. Kaufmann, 1968): (1) that the universe is uniform and permanent, and (2) that the laws to be discovered about the development of organisms are all absolute ones, whether they involve variables lying inside or outside the organism. Although sampling and technological considerations limit science to generating probabilistic laws, these probabilistic statements are regarded as unbiased estimates of absolute ones (Hempel, 1966).

Alternatively, a contextual paradigm assumes: (1) *constant change* of all levels of analysis, and (2) *embeddedness* of each level with all others, the idea that changes in one promote changes in all. The assumption of constant change means that there is no complete uniformity or constancy. Rather than change being a to-be-explained phenomenon, a perturbation in a stable system, change is a given (Overton, 1978); thus, the task of the scientist is to describe, explain, and optimize the parameters and trajectory of processes (i.e., variables that show time-related changes in their quantity and/or quality).

This brings us to the second assumption of contextualism, which stresses the interrelation of all levels of analysis. Because phenomena are not seen as static, but rather as change processes, and because any change process occurs within a similarly (i.e., constantly) changing world (of processes), any target change must be conceptualized in the context of the other changes within which it is embedded. Thus, change will constantly continue as a consequence of reciprocal interactions among embedded levels, and thus we arrive at the idea of dynamic interaction, as well as multilevel embeddedness.

Implications for probabilistic-epigenetic and life-span views of development. Overton (in press) has explained that conceptualizations of human development consistent with a contextual viewpoint are not incompatible with those that stress the organized and active organism (e.g., Schneirla, 1957). Indeed, as noted earlier, Overton (in press) believes that the merger of organicism and contextualism – in what he terms organismic contextualism – constitutes the paradigm for the life-span view of human development, a view which, in present terms, seeks to understand the systematic, reciprocal relations across life between an organized and active organism and an organized and active context. In fact, in Schneirla's (1957) specification of the analytic agenda for the study of behavioral development (cited in Chapter 1), his first three points stress the organized, developmental, and multilevel processes of the active organism, while the fourth point emphasizes that the first three are embedded in, and must be understood in the context of, the prevailing developmental context.

In other words, what we here label a contextual view of human development is not distinct from the conception labeled by Overton (in press) as organismic–contextual; in turn, these positions are, in the present view, isomorphic with the probabilistic-epigenetic position introduced by Baldwin and Poulton (1902), developed by Maier and Schneirla (1935) and Schneirla (1957), and elaborated by Gottlieb (1970, 1976a, 1976b) as well as other developmentalists (Gollin, 1981; Scarr, 1982; Scarr & McCartney, 1983). For instance, Scarr and McCartney propose a concept of genotype influencing environment wherein there exists

a *probabilistic* connection between a person and the environment. It is more likely that people with certain genotypes will receive certain kinds of parenting, evoke certain responses from others, and select certain aspects from the available environments [Belsky, in press; Kendall et al., in press; Lerner, 1982]; but nothing is rigidly determined. The idea of genetic differences, on the other hand, has seemed to imply to many that the person's developmental fate was preordained without regard to experience. This is absurd. By invoking the idea of genotype → environment effects, we hope to emphasize a probabilistic connection between genotypes and their environments. (Scarr & McCartney, 1983, p. 428; bracketed references added)

Thus, according to the contextual view (Overton, in press), the systematically organized organism constrains, delimits, or simply affects the context that affects it (Baldwin & Poulton, 1902; Lerner, 1978, 1979, 1982; Lerner & Busch-Rossnagel, 1981; Mischel, 1977; Schneirla, 1957; Snyder, 1981); in short, contextualism is not used in its ''pure'' form, that is, as a paradigm that stresses the dispersive nature of life (Pepper, 1942). Instead, it is merged with organicism – in ways specified by Schneirla (1957) and by Gottlieb (1970) – in order to address the problems of understanding how multiple change processes, those of an organism and of a multilevel context, combine to provide the probabilistic-epigenetic character of development (e.g., see Gollin, 1981; Gottlieb, 1970; Lerner, 1978, 1979; Meacham, 1976, 1977; Riegel, 1975). While a personological explanation of human development is therefore seen as quite limited from this perspective (Baltes et al., 1980), this view does not mean *only* that the individual's ontogeny must be understood as linked to his or her family and society. In addition, it means that the inner and outer syntheses that comprise the human condition have to be integrated as well; biological and cultural change, or in other words biocultural, historical, or evolutionary changes, must be understood (Baltes et al., 1980; Lerner, 1978; Lewontin & Levins, 1978; Schneirla, 1959; Tobach & Schneirla, 1968).

As an illustration of how the view of developmental processes promoted by organismic contextualism may be seen as consistent with the components of probabilistic epigenesis discussed in Chapter 1, we may consider Gollin's (1981) statement that

the relationships between organisms and environments are not interactionist, as interaction implies that organism and environment are separate entities that come together at an interface. Organism and environment constitute a single life process.... For analytic convenience, we may treat various aspects of a living system and various external environmental and biological features as independently definable properties. Analytical excursions are an essential aspect of scientific inquiry, but they are hazardous if they are primarily reductive. An account of the *collective behavior* of the parts as an organized entity is a necessary complement to a reductive analytic program, and serves to restore the information content lost in the course of the reductive excursion.... In any event, the relationships that contain the sources of change are those between organized systems and environments, not between heredity and environment. (Gollin, 1981, p. 231–2).

A similar view has been expressed by Baltes (1979b), but in regard to the life-span perspective:

Life-span developmental psychologists emphasize *contextualistic–dialectic* paradigms of development (Datan & Reese, 1977; Lerner, Skinner, & Sorell, 1980; Riegel, 1976) rather than the use of "mechanistic" or "organismic" ones more typical of child development work. There are two primary rationales for this preference. One is, of course, evident also in current child development work. As development unfolds, it becomes more and more apparent that individuals act on the environment and produce novel behavior outcomes, thereby making the active and selective nature of human beings of paramount importance. Furthermore, the recognition of the interplay between age-graded, history-graded, and non-normative life events suggests a contextualistic and dialectical conception of development. This dialectic is further accentuated by the fact that individual development is the reflection of multiple forces which are not always in synergism, or convergence, nor do they always permit the delineation of a specific set of endstates. (P. 2)

Conclusions. The merger of contextualism and organicism is associated with the life-span ideas of embeddedness and dynamic interaction and with the probabilistic-epigenetic position that human biology is both a producer *and* a product of social and cultural change (cf. Scarr, 1982); thus, organismic contextualism is a position that contrasts with those of other scholars who, in writing about the relation between biological and social change, stress either that the former is primarily the unidirectional shaper of the latter (Wilson, 1975) or that the two are relatively independent (Campbell, 1975). The organismic–contextual ideas found in the life-span view and in the probabilistic-epigenetic conceptualization of development lead to the position that any level of analysis may be understood in the context of the biological, cultural, and ontogenetic changes of which it is a part (Tobach, 1978; Toulmin, 1981) and that the idea of "one level in isolation" as the "prime mover" of change is not a useful one. Conceptual and empirical support for these interpretations of the implications of embeddedness will be presented throughout the following chapters.

If change at multiple interrelated levels of analysis characterizes the human life span, then neither specific ontogenetic outcomes (Baltes, 1979b) nor totally uniform features of development at any phase of ontogeny necessarily characterize the life course (Toulmin, 1981). Instead, a human life span is characterized by the potential for individual flexibility as a consequence of multilevel, embedded plastic processes (Maier & Schneirla, 1935; Schneirla, 1957; Tobach & Schneirla, 1968), and human lives may differ in the incidence of flexibility because of interindividual differences in the progression of plastic processes.

In sum, because of a superordinate consistency with an organismic–contextual paradigm (Overton, in press), the ideas associated with the probabilistic-epigenetic view of development converge with those associated with the life-span perspective, and together they suggest that dynamic interactions among multiple, embedded levels of analysis provide a basis for human plasticity. As noted above, however, the key propositions associated with a life-span perspective may not only be discussed insofar as they are associated with an organismic-contextual paradigm; in turn, the propositions may be discussed in regard to a set of interrelated implications derived from them. Although these implications have been implied above, it is useful to address them explicitly.

Implications of the propositions

To briefly recapitulate the import of the two key assumptions of the life-span perspective, let me note that the ideas of embeddedness and dynamic interactionism together mean that, first, individual developmental phenomena occur in the context of the developmental and nondevelopmental change phenomena of other levels of analysis; and, second, that developments or changes on one level influence and are influenced by developments or changes at these other levels. There are at least three major implications of the ideas of embeddedness and dynamic interactionism:

1. *The potential for plasticity.* The idea that changes at one level are reciprocally dependent on changes at other levels suggests that there is always some possibility for altering the status of a variable or process at any given level of analysis. Simply put, the character of the interaction among levels of analysis means that there is a potential to change the functioning of any target level (or target variable) and indeed of the system of interlevel relations itself.

Nevertheless, this potential for plasticity is not construed by life-span developmentalists to mean that there are no limits on change. By virtue of its structural organization a system delimits the range of changes it may undergo (Brent, in press); such a structural constraint holds for any level of analysis. For example, the prior developmental organization of a system constrains the potential of a later influence to effect a change in the system as easily as would have been the case if that same influence acted earlier in development (Lerner, 1978, 1979; Schneirla, 1957).

That phenomena at one point in life may influence later functioning is summarized by life-span developmentalists in the concept of *developmental embeddedness* (Parke, R. D., pers. comm., December 1982). Life-span developmentalists emphasize that one must consider not only the changes across life but the constancies as well. Indeed, as indicated in Chapter 1, a key issue within the life-span perspective is to understand the relation between processes that serve to promote constancy and those that serve to promote change (e.g., see Lerner, 1976). That is, and again to recall the orthogenetic principle of Werner (1957), life-span development is concerned with understanding the developmental syntheses between continuous and discontinuous processes (Lerner, 1978, 1979).

Nevertheless, despite their acknowledgment of limits and constraints on change and their emphasis on the concept of developmental embeddedness, life-span developmentalists take the notion of a potential for plasticity to mean that the system is never necessarily completely limited or constrained (Brim & Kagan, 1980) and that as a consequence of the dynamic interaction among multiple levels of analysis means may be found to reorganize or restructure a system, even in advanced periods of that system's development (Baltes & Baltes, 1980; Baltes et al., 1980; Greenough & Green, 1981).

Many life-span developmentalists might agree with geneticist R. C. Lewontin's (1981) views about the issue of constraints:

It is trivially true that material conditions of one level constrain organization at higher levels *in principle*. But that is not the same as saying that such constraints are quantitatively nontrivial. Although every object in the universe has a gravitational interaction with every other object, no matter how distant, I do not, in fact, need to adjust my body's motion to the movement of individuals in the next room. The question is not whether the nature of the human genotype is relevant to social organization, but whether the former constrains the latter in a nontrivial way, or whether the two levels are *effectively* decoupled. It is the claim of vulgar sociobiology that some kinds of human social organization are either impossible, or that they can be maintained only at the expense of constant psychic and political stress, which will inevitably lead to undesirable side effects because the nature of the human genome dictates a "natural" social organization. Appeals to abstract dependencies (in principle) of one level or another do not speak to the concrete issue of whether society is genetically constrained in an important way.

 . . . in fact, constraints at one level may be destroyed by higher level activity. No humans can fly by flapping their arms because of anatomical and physiological constraints that reflect the human genome. But humans do fly, by using machines that are the product of social organization and that could not exist without very complex social interaction and evolution. As another example, the memory capacity of a single individual is limited, but social organization, through written records and the complex institutions associated with them, makes all knowledge recoverable for each individual. Far from being constrained by lower-level limitations, culture transcends them and feeds back to lower levels to relieve the constraints. Social organization, and human culture in particular, are best understood as negating constraints rather than being limited by them. (P. 244)

2. *The person as a producer of his or her own development.* A second implication of the two key propositions of the life-span perspective is that it is possible to view variables from any level of analysis as an influence on variables from the other levels. From the perspective of individual psychological development, this means that a person may affect the context that affects him or her, in essence providing feedback to him- or herself.

In other words, the individual helps produce his or her own development (Lerner, 1982; Lerner & Busch-Rossnagel, 1981; Scarr & McCartney, 1983) – by constituting a distinct stimulus to others (e.g., through characteristics of physical or behavioral individuality), through his or her capabilities as a processor of the world (e.g., in regard to cognitive structure and mode of emotional reactivity), through active behavioral agency (Bakan, 1966; Block, 1973), and, ultimately the most flexible means, by behaviorally shaping or selecting his or her contexts (Kendall, Lerner, & Craighead, in press; Mischel, 1977; Snyder, 1981). The life-span emphasis on the individual as producer of his or her own development leads to a focus on processes of self-regulation, control, and self-efficacy.

3. *The potential for intervention.* The potential for plasticity implies that means may be found to prevent, ameliorate, or enhance undesired or nonvalued developments or behaviors (cf. Baltes & Danish, 1980) using a multidisciplinary approach. In addition, the idea of developmental embeddedness suggests that one may take a historical approach to intervention, and for instance devise long-term preventative strategies (Lerner & Ryff, 1978). However, individual ontogeny is not the only aspect of history that may be considered here. Life-span developmentalists appreciate the features of intergenerational transmission (e.g., see Bengtson & Troll, 1978); they envision the possibility of intervention with future parents to prevent undesired outcomes in yet-to-be-conceived offspring. I will return to this point later in the book, but an example that may be given here is of the possibility of changing the type of birth control precautions of sexually active young adolescents in order to prevent the conception and birth of a child consequently at risk for several health problems as a consequence of being born to a young adolescent mother.

Finally in regard to the implications of the life-span perspective for intervention, let me emphasize that the view that there is a potential for plasticity across life does not mean one should ignore or not invest in treating problems in early life. Rather, the life-span perspective incorporates the ideas that there are always constraints on change and that plasticity is not equipotential across life; that is, while plasticity may be considered ubiquitous, its potential for actualization operates within an increasingly narrower range of structures and functions with time (cf. Baltes & Baltes, 1980; Clarke & Clarke, 1976; Greenough & Green, 1981). Thus, intervention may be more appropriate early in life, when the system is being organized and there may be fewer constraints on its ability to change. Nevertheless, even if early intervention is not possible, according to the life-span perspective there may still be means, albeit more difficult ones, to effect desired change.

Conclusions

I will return at several places in this book to these life-span views about the possibility for intervening across life. Here, it is useful to make three points about the present status of the life-span perspective. First, in studying the complex interrelations among organism and context, life-span developmentalists (e.g., Baltes, 1968; Schaie, 1965) employ particular types of research designs and methodologies (e.g., sequential designs, multivariate statistics, cohort analysis). Second, they seek both methodological and substantive collaboration with scholars from disciplines traditionally unrelated (or only tangentially related) to individual psychological or personological studies – for example, life-course sociology (e.g., Brim, 1966, 1968; Brim & Kagan, 1980; Brim & Ryff, 1980; Elder, 1974, 1979; Riley, 1978, 1979). Third, the initial impetus for these methodological and multidisciplinary activities were conceptual considerations. If contextual influences were not seen as crucial for understanding individual development, then neither methods for their assessment in relation to the individual nor information about the character of their analysis would have been undertaken.

In sum, the development of life-span development psychology in the 1970s has been associated with renewed interest in a multidisciplinary view of human development. This view suggests that individual changes across life both produce and are produced within multiple levels of context; the view thus rests on a conception of development that may be described as contextual (Pepper, 1942). To the extent that context provides a basis for development, then, individuals may be seen as producers of their development. Moreover, the very nature of human plasticity suggests ways in which multidisciplinary research and intervention efforts can enhance human functioning. In the following chapters I hope to provide support for this view by discussing research at several levels of analysis. The discussion, which encompasses areas ranging from the molecular to the molar, begins in the next chapter by focusing on recent research pertinent to gene therapy.

3 Gene marking, recombinant DNA technology, and gene transfer: toward true gene therapy

Are human genetic processes sufficiently plastic to permit the development of intraindividual flexibility? Before addressing this question it is useful to consider how thoroughly human genetic endowment ensures systematic interindividual differences. Our genetic endowment provides a basis of the uniqueness of each human life and provides substance to the claim that all humans have a unique heredity–environment interactive history (Hirsch, 1970; Lerner, 1976, 1978, 1979; McClearn, 1981). Estimates of the number of gene pairs in humans typically range between 10,000 and 100,000 (Bodmer & Cavalli-Sfarza, 1976; Stern, 1973), and if one considers how much genotypic variability can be produced by the reshuffling process of meiosis occurring with 100,000 gene pairs, then the potential for variability is so enormous that "it is next to impossible that there have ever been two individuals with the same combination of genes" (McClearn, 1981, p. 19).

Indeed, Hirsch (1970) conservatively estimates that there are over 7×10^{17} (70 trillion) potential human genotypes. Bodmer and Cavalli-Sforza (1976) estimate that each human has the capacity to generate any one of 10^{3000} different eggs or sperm; by comparison, their estimate of the number of sperm of all men who have ever lived is only 10^{24}. Thus, considering

10^{3000} possible eggs being generated by an individual woman and 10^{3000} possible sperm being generated by an individual man, the likelihood of anyone ever – in the past, present, or future – having the same genotype as anyone else (excepting multiple identical births, of course) becomes dismissably small (McClearn, 1981, p. 19).

A given human's genetic individuality may be seen to be even greater if we recognize that *genetic* does not mean *congenital*, that is, that the "total genome is not functioning at fertilization, or at birth, or at any other time of life" (McClearn, 1981, p. 26); the expression of any individual human genotype is a developmental phenomenon, influenced in regard to the turning on and/or off of genes by the endogenous and the exogenous components of the individual's genotype–environment interaction history (Jacob & Monod, 1961; McClearn, 1970, 1981; Schaie, Anderson, McClearn, & Money, 1975). For instance,

33

McClearn (1981, p. 26) gives the illustration of "the differential production of certain kinds of hemoglobin during various phases of development. For example, production of the beta chain accelerates at the time of birth and peaks after a few months, whereas production of the alpha chain rises prenatally and maintains a high level."

A still further indication of the possible variability among humans is the nature of genes' molecular structure: The estimated 6 billion nucleotide bases that comprise the DNA of the human genome (McClearn, 1981) provide an enormous "population" within which mutation – permanent alterations in genetic material – can occur.

Interindividual variability can be traced not only to the molecular structure of the gene, however, but also to genes' functional characteristics. These functional features, which we shall now consider, constitute the genetic components of human plasticity; they provide the basis of intraindividual change.

Genotype "fluidity" and gene transfer

Advances in genetic chemistry (often termed molecular biology) have revealed that genes, which control the formation of proteins and enzymes (Berg, 1981), are open to both proximal and distal contextual influences and can in fact be manipulated in vitro and, more recently, in vivo. Thus, genes are appropriate targets of intervention. A proximal contextual influence in a gene is illustrated by effects produced by other genes, that is, by gene interactions. Distal contextual influences are those produced by effects of the extra-organism environment. For instance, Uphouse and Bonner (1975) assessed the transcription to DNA by RNA from the brains or livers of rats exposed to either high environmental enrichment (i.e., living in a cage with eleven other rats and having "toys" and mazes available for exploration), low environmental enrichment (i.e., living in a cage with one other rat but no exploration materials), or isolation (i.e., living in a cage alone and with no exploration materials). The RNA from the brains for the environmentally enriched rat showed a level of transcription of DNA significantly greater than that of the other groups. No significant differences were found with liver RNA. Grouse, Schrier, Bennett, Rosenzweig, and Nelson (1978) also found significant differences between the brain RNA of rats reared in environmentally rich versus environmentally impoverished contexts. In addition, Grouse, Schrier, and Nelson (1979) found that the total RNA complexity of brain RNA was greater for normally sighted kittens than for kittens who had both eyelids sutured upon birth. However, the RNAs from the nonvisual cortices and from subcortical structures were not different for the two groups. Grouse et al. conclude that the normal development of the visual cortex, which is dependent on visual experience, involves a greater amount of genetic expression than occurs in the absence of visual experience. Given such findings about the contextual modifiability of genetic material, it is possible to assert that genes are appropriate targets of intervention.

As further support for this view, Lewin (1981a, 1981b, 1982e) cites abundant evidence that the gene's DNA structure is markedly fluid, that genes and other genetic elements have surprising mobility within a genome. For instance, genomes of plants, sea urchins, or even more complex organisms reveal indisputable evidence of DNA sequence amplification and rearrangement.

At a less sophisticated level of genetic organization than humans, in prokaryotic (nonnucleated) cells, there is now evidence for the existence of transposable genetic elements, *transposons*, which may be defined (Kleckner, 1981) as "genetic entities...capable of inserting as discrete, nonpermuted DNA segments at many different sites in prokaryotic genomes...[and promoting] other types of DNA rearrangements...mechanistically related to transposition" (pp. 341–2).

Kleckner notes that while it is certain that "transposable elements in prokaryotic organisms are widespread, diverse, and highly evolved in both mechanistic and regulatory properties" (1981, p. 343), there remain unanswered questions about the transposition process and about the evolutionary bases of transposons. Thus: "transposons may have evolved as nature's tools for genetic engineering," or the existence of transposons may instead be "attributable solely to their ability to overreplicate the host; their ability to replicate and move would permit them to escape the normal mechanisms which could eliminate DNA sequences for which no direct phenotype selection exists" (Kleckner, 1981, p. 343).

In Chapter 6 we will return to a discussion of overreplication of genetic elements, when we consider the potential links among such molecular genetic processes and micro- and macroevolution. Here, however, we should note that the presence and functional character of transposable elements in prokaryotes serve to discredit the notion of a fixed genotype established at conception. Conversely, the notion of a fluid genome – in which there is a constant flux of sequences – is today an accepted fact (Lewin, 1981a); that is, "the existence of a range of mechanisms beyond classic [genetic] recombination, that can cause heritable rearrangements of genetic material" (Lewin, 1982e, p. 42) is now firmly established.

Recent evidence of genetic mobility indicates that genes can "jump" across species' barriers, even in higher organisms. For example, Benveniste and Todaro (1982) report that

retroviral genes can be transferred under *natural conditions* between distantly related mammals, incorporated into their germ lines, and be subsequently inherited as cellular genes. The first example showed that the baboon type C viruses...were incorporated into the germ line of cats, where they are present in 10 to 50 copies per haploid genome, and are inherited in the same Mendelian fashion as other cellular genes. (P. 1202)

The authors further speculate [p. 1202] that "these viruses and other extrachromosomal elements...may provide some of the genetic plasticity that is being increasingly revealed among eukaryotes [nucleated cells]."

The plasticity of eukaryotic genes has been usefully exploited by a "succession of increasingly specialized techniques for bringing together in a single cell nuclear and cytoplasmic elements from dissimilar parent cells" (Graf, 1982, p. 496). Such *gene transformation* or *gene transfer* presently constitutes "an experimental process for modifying the heritable genotypic and phenotypic content of a cell by causing the cell to take up and to express gene sequences of purified DNA that has been isolated from donor cells" (Graf, 1982, p. 496).

Gene transfer thus provides the means for identifying genes of a given family and analyzing the functions of gene molecules (Goodenow et al., 1982, p. 679). For instance, McKnight and Kingsbury (1982) have developed a technique for studying gene function which involves introducing clusters of mutations into DNA at specific locations. Then, as Marx (1982b) points out, by "constructing a series of mutants in which the position of the...mutant is systematically moved, researchers can rapidly scan a length of DNA to see which regions are critical for the activities or the protein product of a gene, or...which regions are involved in regulating gene expression" (p. 434).

To illustrate these techniques we may note that Hood and his colleagues (e.g., Goodenow, McMillan, Örn, Nicolson, Davidson, Frelinger, & Hood, 1982; Moore, Sher, Sun, Eakle, & Hood, 1982) combined the techniques of gene transfer, gene cloning (replication), and gene sequence analysis (specification of the amino acid sequences of a gene) to investigate the mouse's *major histocompatability complex* (MHC) – the set of genes that controls many of the activities of immune cells. These researchers were able to establish that a specific mouse gene that encodes a particular chemical (a polypeptide) is involved in the production of a key antigen, that is, a key component of the mouse's immune system. Thus, the activities of such genes, in particular "the role of their products in mediating the myriad interactions between immune cells" (Marx, 1982a, p. 400), can now be assessed directly, and it is reasonable to believe that "in the future, other...functional genes will be defined by the strategies of gene cloning, gene transfer, and sequence analysis" (Moore et al., 1982, p. 682). Commenting on the implications of this work, Hood (in Marx, 1982a, p. 400) notes that "this is the first system for which we can study cell–cell recognition at the molecular level" and predicts that future experiments in this area "will revolutionize cellular immunology."

The success to date of such techniques relies on the plasticity of eukaryotic genetic matter; thus, rather than there being a gene for plasticity (Wilson, 1975), genes, their components, and their processes as well are plastic.

For example, although only 1 percent of the human genome has been mapped, it is already possible to palliate some genetic diseases pharmacologically or by environmental manipulation, and in the near future the antenatal repair of a flawed genome may be possible (McKusick, 1981). One example of such possible future interventions relates to the rapid advancements being made in determining how plasma cholesterol is regulated by lipoprotein receptors. Brown, Kovanen, and Goldstein (1981) report that the lipoprotein transport system holds the key to understanding the mechanisms by which genes, hormones, and human dietary habits interact to regulate the plasma cholesterol level in humans. Crucial components of this system are lipoprotein receptors in liver and other tissues, which mediate the uptake and degradation of cholesterol-carrying lipoproteins. The number of lipoprotein receptors, and hence the efficiency of disposal of plasma cholesterol, can be increased by cholesterol-lowering drugs. Regulation of lipoprotein receptors thus can be maintained pharmacologically in the therapy of human hypercholesterolemia and atherosclerosis.

Examples of McKusick's (1981) point about the potential for antenatal repair of a flawed genome currently rest in two interrelated areas of research, one pertaining to the study of the intrinsic DNA-repair systems (Howard-Flanders, 1981), a second to the study of gene control. Obviously, research in the first area (intrinsic DNA-repair systems) involves studying processes by which genes and the enzymes they produce turn on and off – control – their repair processes. What distinguishes the second line of research is its emphasis on recombinant DNA technology for gene replacement (discussed in a later section).

A key problem with regard to gene control is that, while it is clear that genes turn on and off as the organism develops and adapts to contextual conditions (Ptashne, Johnson, & Pabo, 1982), due to the difficulty in studying such gene regulation in the complex cells of higher organisms, relatively little information about the precise features of gene regulation has been uncovered in such cells. Research has thus focused on the relatively simpler task of studying gene regulation in bacteria, where important discoveries have been made. For instance, Ptashne et al. (1982) have delineated the molecular mechanisms that switch lambda virus genes on and off in particular strains of the *Escherichia coli.*

Howard-Flanders (1981), commenting on the study of intrinsic DNA-repair systems, notes that whereas cellular DNA, whether bacterial or human, is quite sensitive to damage (e.g., by harmful radiation or chemical agents in the environment), the stability and precision of replication of DNA are maintained by enzymes that continually repair genetic lesions. Although numerous instances of DNA-repair systems have been studied for several years, only since about 1979 have the precise details of the regulatory processes involved in these repair systems become known. As the DNA-repair systems have become better understood and thus amenable to experimental manipulation, increasing evidence has indicated that (1) DNA damage and its repair are significant factors in the etiology and remission of human cancer and in the process of aging; and (2) the potential exists for devising means of intervention to alter disease and other processes (Howard-Flanders, 1981).

Gene marking

Scientists have begun to locate individual genes on human chromosomes and are making great strides toward reconstructing the nucleotide sequences of the genes themselves (McKusick, 1981).

However, as with the study of DNA-repair systems, generally useful techniques for the specification of these sequences have been developed only relatively recently (Sanger, 1981). The difficulty in obtaining accurate complete descriptions of these sequences is attributable to the large size of DNA molecules. The *smallest* DNA molecule contains about 5000 base pairs (Sanger, 1981). Initially, work on the determination of nucleotide sequences was conducted in some relatively small RNA molecules – transfer RNAs each consisting of about 75 nucleotides (Sanger, 1981).

The recent advances in sequence determination have used various instances of the enzyme DNA polymerase (which copies single-stranded DNA). For example, Kunkel and Loeb (1981) determined the fidelity of copying natural DNA in vitro with each of three classes of mammalian, eukaryotic DNA polymerases. Although one of the tested DNA polymerases was superior to the others in terms of accuracy of copying, the error rates of all tested polymerases were much greater than those of in vivo DNA replicative processes. This indicates that the DNA polymerases had not copied all the genes, and their associated enzymes, involved in the above-discussed DNA-repair systems.

Despite such limitations, there have been notable successes. Reddy, Smith, and Aaronson (1981), for instance, report that the complete nucleotide sequence of a mammalian transforming retrovirus, Moloney murine sarcoma virus, has been determined. O'Brien and Nash (1982) have constructed a genetic map of 31 biochemical loci on 17 syntenic (linkage) groups of the domestic cat. Moreover, Berg (1981) observes that mapping and – as will be discussed in more detail below – manipulating, through recombinant DNA methods, the relatively small genomes of such prokaryotic microorganisms as the bacterium *E. coli* (and the viruses that inhabit them) are now routine procedures.

As a consequence of such successful work on gene mapping, which in its last stage involves the assignment of genes to chromosomes, several important insights have been gained about the role of genes in various diseases. For example, advances in gene marking may soon provide a new means for preventive intervention, through counseling, of the inheritance of genetic diseases (Lewin, 1981a). The markers being studied are DNA polymorphisms, genetic loci occupied by one of a group of readily identifiable gene variants, or *alleles* (Lewin, 1981a). Researchers at both MIT and the University of Utah have been able to excise the locus from the genome, analyze its overall structure, and determine which variant it represents. Analysis and identification of only a few hundred of such markers (from among the potentially thousands that may exist in the human genome) will make it possible to begin constructing a map for disease linkage. That is, once the basic complement of markers is ascertained, it will be possible to determine which loci are associated with which others through the processes of meiosis and crossing-over when gametes are formed (Lewin, 1981a). Then, after ascertaining the markers with which the inheritance of each genetic disease is associated, preventative intervention becomes a possibility.

Experimental gene marking has also resulted in the finding that enzymes involved in various metabolic pathways are not, as a rule, syntenic (associated with genes that have the property of being on the same chromosome) and in the discovery of the location of the specific chromosomal sites of about three dozen enzyme defects (errors of metabolism) and other genetic disorders (McKusick, 1981). That is, the particular problematic enzyme, associated with a particular gene from a specific chromosome, in a syntenic metabolic pathway, has been identified in several disorders. Often, with such disorders, methods of recombinant DNA analysis have enabled work in chromosomal anatomy to proceed to a point where the molecular basis for a defect may be identified at the DNA level itself. Let us consider the role of recombinant DNA techniques in this and other related work.

Recombinant DNA technology

The methods collectively known as recombinant DNA techniques derive from the study of gene structure through microbial genetics and DNA biochemistry (Wetzel, 1980). In nature it would be difficult to find a DNA molecule among higher organisms that is not already a recombinant one: Recombination is one of the key mechanisms by which new individuals are generated (Wetzel, 1980). Laboratory recombinant DNA techniques are in vitro versions of these natural phenomena; the techniques consist of purifying and identifying genetic material from one source, manipulating it to make it suitable for insertion into a new host, and isolating a colony of cells possessing the desired new genetic material (Wetzel, 1980).

As indicated earlier, recombinant DNA manipulation of relatively small genomes of prokaryotic organisms such as *E. coli* is now a routine matter (Berg, 1981). And while we cannot yet interpret the instructions contained in the sequence of DNA bases or specify the critical mechanisms of control in any single eukaryotic gene with the molecular detail with which the lac operon of *E. coli*

is understood (Brown, 1981), an "explosive growth" in the application of recombinant DNA methods has provided new insights into the mechanisms of
gene regulation in normal and developmentally interesting animals (Berg, 1981).
For example, there is known to exist an abundance of gene control points and
at least two types of eukaryotic gene control mechanisms: (1) those in which
genes are altered – through domination, amplification, rearrangement, and modification; and (2) those in which *gene expression is modulated* – transcriptional,
posttranscriptional, and translocational control.

Techniques also exist for insertion of DNA into the cells of plants and animals.
For example, in vitro transformed mouse bone marrow cells have established a
viable cell line when returned to mice (Cline, Stang, Mercola, Morse, Ruprecht,
Browne, & Salser, 1980; Wetzel, 1980). When Cline et al. (1980) introduced
a gene that provides resistance to the toxic drug methotrexate into the bone
marrow cells of mice, the treated mice proved more resistant to the drug; and
in a recent experiment by Gordon, Scangos, Plotkin, Barbosa, and Ruddle (in
press), a viral gene injected into mouse embryos and newborn mice retained the
viral DNA sequences in their cells.

At this point our accounts of gene transfer, marking, and mapping and recombinant DNA technology converge to provide a basis for discussing genetic
engineering – specifically, and most important from the standpoint of enhancing
the human condition, gene therapy.

Gene therapy

To use recombinant DNA technology as part of a systematic effort to implement
human gene therapy, one would have to use recombinant DNA methods to
perform genetic manipulations on cells that would be subsequently returned to
the human body. The first steps in this process involve identifying the locus of
the gene defect through genetic mapping techniques and obtaining a supply of
the normal gene in multiple copies (which, as noted, has already been accomplished for a few human genes). The healthy human genes (which for some
proteins involved in genetic diseases have already been isolated and developed),
along with the necessary control elements, would then be inserted into the
chromosome of the defective cell and the altered cell reestablished in the host
organism through "gene surgery" or "gene transplantation" (Wetzel, 1980).
This last step has already been accomplished in laboratory animals (McKusick,
1981). For example Rubin and Spradling (1982) have developed a means of
efficiently transferring specific DNA segments (without rearrangement) into the
germ line of a multicellular organism – the fruit fly (*Drosophila*) – and found
that the transformation was stably inherited in subsequent generations. The intent

of the transformation was to correct a genetic deficit in the host strain, and the defect was indeed eliminated in the transformed flies. Moreover, the stability of the inheritance of the transformation indicated that the genetic deficit could be fully and permanently corrected by the transferred gene.

Among the formidable problems that remain to be solved is how to transform enough cells to normalize the patient's biochemistry – that is, to make sure that the gene is expressed at the right time, that it is linked to the chromosomal mechanisms that normally control it (McKusick, 1981). Moreover, until quite recently most of the progress in gene transfer derived from research done with cultured cells, and while researchers can now transfer practically any isolatable gene into cultured cells, much work needs to be done in the study of the control of gene expression in mammalian, and particularly human, cells (Marx, 1980).

Thus, Anderson and Fletcher (1980) point out that currently we can purify only genes whose products are known and can be isolated, and that we are today dealing only with single genes. Mercola and Cline (1980), two of the researchers involved in the previously cited mice experiments (Cline et al., 1980), are nevertheless optimistic about the potential for identifying, cloning, and inserting genes into humans in order to rectify both genetic and nongenetic disorders. They believe genetic disorders of the blood are a likely successful first target of studies aimed at inserting normal genes in humans. In addition, they believe the technology for cloning appropriate genes and inserting them into marrow cells of patients with Gaucher's disease will be feasible soon.

In the search for ways to make the introduction of functional genes into living animals a routine matter, the intermediate goal of creating new strains of organisms having foreign or systematically altered genes is currently being pursued (Marx, 1982c). Such successful gene transfer and new species creation, it is believed, will lead to a greater understanding of development at the molecular level and, more specifically, of how genes are turned on and off in specific tissues (Marx, 1982c). An example of such research is the work of Beatrice Mintz and her colleagues at the Institute for Cancer Research in Philadelphia, who have provided evidence not only that a foreign gene of a virus can be transferred into a live mammal but that, in addition, it may be possible to create a new strain carrying the foreign gene (Marx, 1981b, 1982). Mintz's work uses recombinant DNA techniques to prepare purified genes in large enough quantities for injection into the recently fertilized eggs of mice. (Eggs are used in order to maximize the probability of getting the foreign gene into all the cells of the mouse.) Mintz and her colleagues injected a recombinant molecule consisting of bacterial plasmid DNA into which the thymidine kinase gene of herpes simplex virus had been introduced (Marx, 1981b). Of the 33 mice treated in this way, 15 percent – a percentage Mintz considers high – retained intact copies of the transferred gene (Marx, 1981b). More importantly, evidence suggested that when the mice reached adulthood the injected genes were integrated into their chromosomes, an obvious necessity if a new strain is to be created.

As another example, Ruddle and Gordon at Yale found that foreign genetic material inserted into mice eggs was retained, although rearranged in form (Marx, 1981b). When three of the mice reached adulthood the inserted gene was found incorporated into their DNA; one of these animals, a female, produced 6 of 10 offspring that carried the foreign DNA in the same form as the mother (Marx, 1981b). Thus, in this case a new strain was created, albeit with a rearranged copy of the gene originally inserted into the mother.

There are over two thousand known human genetic disorders, some of which can be ameliorated but none of which can currently be cured (Anderson & Diacumakos, 1981). Thus the initial, albeit limited, successes of researchers attempting to transfer genes into living mammals and establish viable new strains are reasons for cautious optimism regarding what the near future may hold for intervention. In this regard, Berg (1981), although critical of the great number of implausible scenarios that have been forwarded about the potential of recombinant DNA technology, or genetic engineering, to treat crippling or fatal genetic disorders, believes that there is no doubt that the development and application of recombinant DNA techniques has put us at the threshold of new forms of medicine.

Underscoring such optimism is the fact that two investigators have recently reported that more complex, eukaryotic genes have been inserted into live mammals. Karl Illmensee of the University of Geneva reported that the human insulin gene remained intact in two mouse embryos developed from eggs which had been injected with DNA carrying that gene (Marx, 1981b). More significantly, Thomas Wagner of Ohio University has indicated the successful transfer into mice of a functional rabbit gene for the protein beta-globin and the transmission of this gene, intact, to a second generation of mice (Marx, 1981c).

Conclusions

In sum, true human gene therapy may reasonably be said to lie in the foreseeable future. Advances in gene marking, recombinant DNA technologies, and gene insertion/transfer methods provide a strong basis for this optimistic appraisal. Conceptually, all this work is possible because the gene is a manipulatable entity. Because the chemicals comprising genes and their effects are accessible targets for intervention, they represent a basis for human change and development – a source of liberation of humans from the diseases that affect their well-being. As we move now to more molar levels of analysis, manifestations of human plasticity will be seen, justifying similar conclusions about the potential for intervention aimed at enhancing human life.

4   Neuroanatomical bases of human plasticity

Consideration of the anatomical characteristics of the human brain provides strong support for the plasticity of human developmental processes. As noted in Chapter 1, and as will be discussed in greater detail in a later chapter, data derived from evolutionary biology and comparative psychology indicate that animals differ in the eventual level of behavioral flexibility attained across their ontogeny. These species differences in behavior are related to corresponding species differences in the ratio of association to sensory fibers in the brain that Hebb (1949) terms the A/S ratio. As Thompson (1981) observes, "moving from more primitive to more complex mammals, following the general course of evolution, the amount of cortex relative to the total amount of brain tissue increases in fairly regular proportions" (p. 7); and although "the basic organization of the cortical sensory and motor areas does not appear to differ markedly from rat to human, . . . as one ascends the mammalian scale of evolution, the relative amount of *association cortex* (cortex that is neither sensory nor motor and is concerned with higher or more complex behavioral functions) increases strikingly" (p. 8). Moreover, the primates, and particularly *Homo sapiens*, exhibit "enormous and disproportionate increases in the amount of cerebral cortex" (Thompson, 1981). And among mammals, humans, although they do not have the largest brain masses, exhibit the highest A/S ratio – indeed "the majority of neurons in the human brain are in the cerebral cortex" (Thompson, 1981).

Thompson underscores the implications of these observations in his discussion of the brain's neural connections. In the human brain, he notes, there are approximately 1 trillion neurons, and each single neuron typically engages in 100–1000 synaptic contacts with other neurons. This means that the number of synapses in a human brain is between 10^{14} to 10^{15}, or about 1 quadrillion. Yet the number of *possible* synaptic connections is still greater: "If we assume that each neuron can contact 100 other neurons and then compute all possible combinations among the 10^{12} neurons, we end up with a number that is larger than the total number of atomic particles that compose the entire known universe. . . . as the

44

brain develops, the *possibilities* for connections among neurons are virtually limitless. This. . . suggests that the capacity of the human brain may be almost without limit'' (Thompson, 1981, p. 3). However, even more than its complex circuitry, the structural responsiveness of human neuroanatomy to experiential influence is a telling indicator of the brain's plasticity. Let us consider the ways in which experiential influences illustrate neuroanatomical plasticity.

Brain plasticity and the role of experience

Studies assessing the effects of experience on brain plasticity may be classified into two general categories: (1) studies that adopt the ''experimental lesion method'' and investigate the effects of brain lesions on an organism's nervous system circuitry and on the circuitry's recovery from the experimentally induced ''pathological'' condition (Cotman & Nieto-Sampedro, 1982); and (2) studies that assess the effects of experiences on the nervous systems, where ''experience'' can be electrical stimulation applied to one or more portions of the nervous system or can involve more molar physical environmental and/or social environmental manipulations (Greenough & Green, 1981).

Relevant to both types of studies are the observations of Cotman and Nieto-Sampedro (1982), who reviewed ''the class of plasticities which appear to involve synapse renewal'' (p. 371). These authors conceive of behavioral plasticity as the susceptibility of behavior to modification and posit that such a behavioral attribute enhances an organism's ability to adapt and survive. In Chapter 1, it will be recalled, I used the term *flexibility* to denote this aspect of behavioral plasticity. In turn, Cotman and Nieto-Sampedro note that in recent years several studies have demonstrated that nervous system circuitry is also very plastic (or, flexible, in the terms used in Chapter 1). Referring to mammals (e.g., rodents), they state:

The structural and functional adaptations that contribute to such plasticity are numerous and can be elicited by many different stimuli. Circuitry adaptations range from modifications in existing connections in response to repeated stimuli to the replacement or renewal of synapses induced by surgical *or environmental manipulations.* . . . when synapse replacement is induced by partial denervation it is clear that new synapses replace those lost. . . . *Long-term changes in brain circuitry can also be induced by more subtle perturbations of the organism or of its environment, some of them identical to the stimuli that cause behavioral plasticity.* . . . reactive synaptic growth and synapse renewal are just an extension of the normal operation and maintenance of brain circuits. (Cotman & Nieto-Sampedro, 1982, pp. 371–372; italics added)

Thus, according to the data reviewed by Cotman and Nieto-Sampedro (1982) – data derived from both lesion and experiential studies – the circuitry of the brain at the molecular level (the level of the synapse) shows flexibility as a consequence of lesion-induced stimulation, as a consequence of stimulation from the organism's molar context, *and* as a consequence of "inductive" (Gottlieb, 1976a) behavioral functioning on the part of the organism itself.

Lynch and Gall (1979) cite further evidence that central nervous system development "is not so genetically hard-wired" as might have been imagined – that is, that "the final architecture of the brain reflects interactions between its neuronal and glial constituents as well as between the organism and its environment" (pp. 138–9). Indeed, Coss and Globus (1978), for example, report that cichlid fish deprived of the opportunity to view their own species have fewer dendritic spines and branches on certain tectal interneurons than do fish reared in community tanks; similarly, they report that social stimulation induces localized formation of spines that swell with synaptic activation. Thus, it is not just stimulation per se that seems influential in the development of neurons and neuronal connections; rather, specifically, social stimulation, as for example provided by the opportunity to view conspecifics, seems to be a key facilitator of neuronal development, a point to which we will return below (see also Greenough & Green, 1981).

Consistent with the concept, presented in Chapter 1, that plasticity exists across life, Cotman and Nieto-Sampedro (1982) cite evidence of circuitry flexibility in adult organisms. As noted above, one line of evidence they review pertains to lesion-induced synaptogenesis in adult mammals (e.g., rodents); they note that partial denervation resulting from direct damage to the nervous system is among the "coarser of the stimuli known to induce synapse renewal" and that such stimulation "of a peripheral or central structure causes intact nerve fibers to sprout new endings and form new synapses that replace those lost as a consequence of the lesion" (Cotman & Nieto-Sampedro, 1982, p. 372). In other words, partial denervation appears to represent an experience that promotes in adults the appearance of capabilities that either are not normally expressed or are expressed in a subtler fashion.

Similarly, Lynch and Gall (1979, p. 138) have concluded that "although the most dramatic examples of nervous system flexibility" are "found in immature animals, . . . the intact, mature axon possesses the capacity to form new, functional synaptic connections in partially deafferented sites, and it is likely that they are able to grow new collateral branches under these circumstances." For example, Jackson and Diamond (1981) report that low-threshold mechanosensory cutaneous nerves readily regenerate in adult rats. In addition, Lynch and Gall (1979) point out that glial cells are capable of remarkable transformations – for example, mitosis and migration – and cite strong evidence indicating that the anatomy of glial cells is greatly influenced by environmental stimulation.

Partial denervation stimulates synaptic growth not only in the immediate area of the lesion, but apparently outside the lesioned area as well (Lynch & Gerling, 1981). For example, Rotshenker (1979) experimentally denervated one of the

two cutaneous pectois muscles of frogs, leaving the other muscle and its associated motor nerve intact. Although the two muscles are innervated by separate
motor nerves, after denervation of just one the nerve endings on the muscle of
the opposite side sprouted from 12% to 30% new synapses.

Lynch and Gall (1979) consider studies of lesion-produced synaptogenesis as
constituting a line of research that demonstrates the plasticity of brain structures
by documenting the capacity of axons, following lesions made in a still-devel-
oping system, to deviate from what might have been thought of as genetically
programmed morphology. According to Lynch and Gall, some experimental
procedures reveal that "radically aberrant circuitry will form in the brain" and
that "such circuits really operate" (p. 131). Moreover, studies of deafferentation
of *mature* dendrites have shown the initiation of plastic changes similar to those
seen in the developing animal; that is, "mature dendrites have demonstrated the
capacity to lose and develop dendritic spines in coordination with the loss and
redevelopment of presynaptic contact" (p. 132). Furthermore, studies of the
effects of applying repetitive electrical stimulation to the cortex indicate resulting
increases in dendritic branching, dendritic field, and spine density (Ruttledge et
al., 1974; Ruttledge, 1976) and "suggest that fully mature dendrites retain
extraordinary plasticity, *even in the absence of pathological conditions*" (Lynch
& Gall, 1979; italics added), a point we will see supported below by the research
of Greenough and his colleagues.

Here we should note some specific examples of lesion-induced synaptogenesis.
Zakon and Capranica (1981) found evidence of regeneration three months after
cutting the auditory nerve of the leopard frog. In addition, binaural cells in the
superior olive reestablished well-matched frequency sensitivies, and the specificity of central connectivity of the auditory system was restored. Thus, even
after severe trauma, neurons and their associated processes have the capacity to
sufficiently correct for the physical insults such that the lesion is repaired and
lost function is restored. Similarly, Elliott and Muller (1982) report that functional
synapses in the central nervous system of the leech were accurately regenerated
with normal frequency after severing of axons.

Such regenerative capacity can apparently occur even when neurons are deprived of intrinsic proteins specifically promoting nerve growth – that is, nerve
growth factor (NGF). Campenot (1981) cultured sympathetic neurons from newborn cats for one month or longer in the absence of nonneuronal cells. The
neurons were found to be capable of regenerating neurites after neuritotomy.
Most interestingly, regeneration occurred even after NGF was withdrawn from
the cultures, even though it was less extensive and was limited to a few days
following neuritotomy. Nevertheless, even after 29 days of NGF deprivation,
reintroduction of NGF initiated a resumption of neurite growth.

Wright and Harding (1982) found that mice trained to discriminate between scented and unscented air lost that ability after bilateral olfactory bulb removal but regained it through the subsequent formation of synaptic connections between regenerated primary olfactory neurons and the cortex of the forebrain. Moreover, the acquisition of a second olfactory-mediated task by long-term bulbectomized mice and controls was indistinguishable. The results of Wright and Harding (1982) not only provide evidence for lesion-induced synaptogenesis in mammals, but indicate that functional (behavioral, in this case) features of the organism that are tied to the lesioned area may also be "regenerated."

The best examples of lesion-induced synaptic growth come not from the study of the frog, leech, mouse, or cat, however, but from the study of the hippocampus in the central nervous system (CNS) of the rat, a region of the CNS of particular concern to behavioral scientists because of its fairly strong link to memory functions in animals and humans (Cotman & Nieto-Sampedro, 1982; Kesner & Novak, 1982). While all types of lesions that have been studied induce synaptic growth, and the new synapses completely restore the synaptic input lost following lesion, the results of the rat hippocampal formation research also provide information about the limits of plasticity in adult organisms studied using experimental lesion techniques. First, methodologically, lesions will promote synapse growth only if a sufficient number of afferents are removed. Second, an afferent will reinnervate a denervated area only when the terminal field of the afferent overlaps with that of the lesioned afferent. Third, and most important for inferences about the degree to which plasticity may exist across life, growth evoked by lesioning promotes only *quantitative* increases in relocation of previously present connections; in the adult organism lesion-induced synaptogenesis does not create *qualitatively* different pathways (Cotman & Nieto-Sampedro, 1982).

However, as noted, it is possible to investigate quantitative and qualitative changes in the mature nervous system that may arise in cases where there does not exist such drastic, coarse, and potentially ontogenetically untypical stimuli as are lesions (especially of the experimentally induced type). In this regard, Cotman and Nieto-Sampedro (1982) cite evidence that synapse loss and replacement (i.e., synapse turnover) is a process that occurs continuously in the mature organism. In fact, they note that such "natural" or "spontaneous" synapse turnover – that is, synapse remodeling in the absence of tissue damage – may be evoked by "experience, changes in environment, and the normal physiological activity of the organism" (p. 379).

Examples of such natural synapse turnover can be found within or outside the CNS. Townes-Anderson and Raviola (1976, 1977, 1978) studied synapses involved in the parasympathetic innervation of the ciliary muscle of adult monkeys; about 2% of the synapses were degenerating, while a corresponding percentage were regenerating. Similarly, the CNS of the bipolar sensory neurons of the olfactory system of several species of mammals show a continuous, 10- to 20-

day cycle of synapse degeneration and regeneration (Graziadei & Monti-Graziadei, 1978, 1979). Let us now consider the role of experience in this natural synapse turnover process.

Experience and natural synapse renewal

Here we shall review further evidence that animals, even adult ones, placed into particular environments (i.e., subjected to particular experiential histories) exhibit alterations in features of the cortex, including number and distribution of synapses (for reviews, see, e.g., Cotman & Nieto-Sampedro, 1982; Greenough, 1975; Greenough & Green, 1981; Kandel & Schwartz, 1981; Rosenzweig & Bennett, 1977, 1978). Uylings and colleagues (Uylings, Kypers, Diamond, and Veltman, 1978; and Uylings, Kypers, and Veltman, 1978) transferred 112-day-old (i.e., adult) rats from the standard laboratory cage environment where they had been reared to an enriched environment. The rats were maintained in this new setting for 30 days, after which their brains were compared to (1) as a control for environment, a group of rats who had also lived for 112 days in the standard laboratory environment and who had remained there for an additional 30 days; and (2) as a control for age effects, a group of rats reared in the standard laboratory environment for 112 days. Analysis of the dendritic branching pattern of these groups showed that an increase in the number of terminal segments in several layers of cortical pyramidal cells correlated with environmental enrichment and with greater age. Results similar to those of Uylings' group were reported by Juraska, Greenough, Elliot, Mack, and Berkowitz (1980) in respect to dendritic branching of pyramidal and stellate neurons in the occipital cortex of rats who were reared in social conditions for their first 145 days and were then placed in either an environmentally complex or an isolated condition for 84 days.

Similarly, Volkmar and Greenough (Volkmar and Greenough, 1972; Greenough and Volkmar, 1973) found up to 15% more dendritic material in the pyramidal and stellate neurons of the visual cortex of animals reared in enriched environments than in animals reared in social isolation; in animals reared in laboratory-typical social conditions, the percentage of dendritic material was less than in the enriched group but greater than in the isolated one. Comparable results have been reported by Globus, Rosenzweig, Bennett, and Diamond (1973). Greenough and Green (1981) conclude:

Taken together, these studies demonstrate that the number of connections of a variety of different types of central nervous system neurons depends to a significant degree on the experience of the organism during its development. This plasticity appears to be widespread in the nervous system – in fact it may well be the rule, rather than the exception.... Even cells in the seemingly "hard-wired" regulatory regions of the brain appear to show a form of developmental plasticity. (p. 170)

Such effects of environmental enrichment can be identified in brain areas outside the cerebral cortex as well. Floeter and Greenough (1979) studied the cerebellums of young monkeys reared either in a nonrestricted or isolated environment or in a socially isolated and sensory- and motor-restricted one. In the first group there were changes in their cerebellums comparable to those described above – that is, comparable to that found when the context is experimentally enhanced. Thus, Floeter and Greenough's data, when seen in the context of the environmental enrichment data, permit the inference that not only does the brain remain available into adulthood for change by enriched and/or special environments, but also that experiences that fall within the range normatively or naturally occurring for the organism promote brain changes. In other words, it may be that brain changes in response to environmental stimulation are a typical part of organisms' lives.

However, here we should recall our discussion (in Chapter 1) of plasticity as a "double-edged sword" – that is, plasticity implies openness to influences that can alter the organism's attributes for better *or* for worse. This can be seen in experiential regimens that, by deactivating parts of the nervous system (in particular the visual and somatosensory systems), adversely influence developmental plasticity in the mature organism (Cotman & Nieto-Sampedro, 1982). Several studies demonstrate that altered levels of usage in these systems can induce circuitry adjustments. For example, Archer, Dubin, and Stark (1982) silenced the action potentials in one eye of neonatal kittens (through intraocular injections of tetrodotoxin). After the drug wore off, an examination of the receptive field properties of individual relay cells in the lateral geniculate nucleus indicated extremely abnormal retinogeniculate synaptic connections. Archer et al. thus concluded that lack of action potential activity leads to abnormal development in the CNS.

In another study monocular deprivation accompanied by artificially induced temporary paralysis resulted in substantial changes in the visual cortex cells of young (four-week-old) kittens, even when monocular deprivation was relatively brief (Freeman & Bonds, 1979). Similarly, Sengelaub and Finlay (1981) found that although there is normally a substantial loss of cells from the retinal ganglion layer of the hamster eye in the first two weeks of postnatal life, if one eye is lost at birth, cell death is reduced in the remaining eye. The authors believe this finding may account for the increased ipsilateral projection from the remaining eye to the thalamus and midbrain found in these organisms.

On the basis of such evidence Greenough and Green (1981, pp. 161–3) point out:

In higher mammals such as rats, cats, and monkeys, visual experience appears to be necessary to the development of a normally functioning visual system....there are fewer synapses on neurons in the visual cortex of animals that have been deprived of vision....for example...mice reared in the dark had fewer spines...on the neurons in [the] visual cortex than did light-reared animals. An even more important type of change may involve the pattern of synaptic connections....dendrites...of some types of neurons were positioned differently in the visual cortex of dark-reared rodents relative to light-reared controls....Similarly...the axons of neurons connected to the deprived eye in monocularly deprived monkeys were constrained to a relatively small area while those connected to the experienced eye were expanded, relative to the pattern in the normally reared cat.

In sum, normative developmental patterns may involve changes in brain anatomy in response to variations in experiential history. However, such flexibility need not always involve salutary outcomes for an organism. The challenge for research is to determine what sorts of experiences lead to what, if any, sorts of changes in what portions of the brain of particular organisms and *at which points in development*. It may be that the effects of experience on the brain are not identical across ontogeny. Let us now consider this issue.

Developmental and age effects and constraints on plasticity

Perhaps the most complete and balanced assessment of age-associated limits on the effects of experience on brain changes has been presented by Greenough (1975; Greenough & Green, 1981), from whose laboratory come some of the best and most recent evidence on adult neuronal plasticity in nonlesioned, nonpathological situations. Greenough and Green (1981) contrast a traditional view of experience and the changing brain with one that has derived from the results of their own research (e.g., Chang & Greenough, 1982; Greenough, Juraska, & Volkmar, 1979; Juraska et al., 1980; West & Greenough, 1972) and that of others (e.g., Rosenzweig, Bennett, & Diamond, 1972a, 1972b). Greenough and Green note:

A simple statement of contemporary thought regarding brain development over the human life-span suggests that the brain goes through three stages. During the initial stage of relatively rapid development, the brain appears uniquely receptive to certain experiences at certain times; in the adult stage, the brain retains its capacity to store information from the environment, but the effects of specific experiences are considerably less profound than during early development; in the stage of aging (which may, in fact, begin quite early) the brain becomes increasingly less capable of directing many kinds of mental and physical performance, and the ability to store and retain information from the environment gradually (or sometimes precipitously) declines.

Rather striking differences in the manner in which the brain interacts with experience during these three stages have led to the postulation that different biological mechanisms are operative. The developing brain is thought to exhibit a very high degree of plasticity or ability to change in the face of experience, which is reflected in anatomical and physiological as well as behavioral measures. The adult brain is thought of as relatively stable from an anatomical and physiological point of view, and information storage as a relatively minor process in terms of the metabolic activity of the brain as a whole (although the assumption by many investigators that metabolic consequences of a single training experience may be discovered suggests an expectation of relatively major involvement of the brain at least for short periods).

The aging brain has been seen to decline in terms of anatomical, physiological, and metabolic as well as behavioral measures, and it has been widely assumed that this relatively inevitable physiological decay underlies the decline of behavioral performance. Thus the developing brain has been viewed as relatively dynamic, adding to its structures and potential; the adult brain as relatively stable; and the aging brain as again dynamic, in the reverse direction, irrevocably declining at rates that apparently vary widely across individuals.

Recently, experimental evidence has begun to challenge these views. First, it has become quite clear that degeneration, including both loss of cells and elimination of cellular processes, is inherent in normal development. Thus, early development is not merely a process of adding to the structure of the brain. Second, there is increasing evidence that the adult brain may remain remarkably plastic from an anatomical perspective. That is, experience appears to continue to modulate the structure of the brain and its cellular components. Third, there is a limited amount of evidence that suggests that the aging brain may retain a considerable degree of flexibility in structure. Although the evidence is far from complete, we can begin to speculate that the structure (and correspondingly the function) of the brain at any point may reflect the historical and current state of a dynamic interplay of growth and degeneration of neuronal processes, with the relative weight of the degeneration aspect increasing in the older years.

This model suggests somewhat different mechanisms whereby experience affects the brain during early development and also suggests that experience may continue to affect the brain in much the same way throughout life. If so, the organism's experience may play an important role in the aging process. (Greenough & Green, 1981, pp. 159–60)

In other words, neuronal loss and renewal can occur across life, or – as emphasized by Riley (1979a) – development and aging are lifelong processes, plasticity of the brain is evident in adulthood, and experience moderates this plasticity.

Although much of the evidence for functional and anatomical plasticity derives from research on young organisms, the points made by Greenough and Green regarding these life-span features of plasticity are not without substantial support. Indeed, other reviewers of the literature (e.g., Black, 1982; Lynch & Gall, 1979; Lynch & Gerling, 1981) and those who have recently reported research (e.g., Bayer, Yackel, & Puri, 1982) reach similar conclusions.

For example, Nottebohm has conducted studies of song learning in adult canaries (e.g., Nottebohm, 1981), work that serves as a good model for studying the brain's plasticity and potential for repair in adulthood (Marx, 1982b). Nottebohm (1981) finds that mature male canaries can learn new song repertoires and that this functional plasticity appears to be underlain by marked anatomical changes, changes that covary with the season of the year. Nottebohm reports that two telecephalic song control nuclei – the hyperstriatum ventrale, pars caudale – and the nucleus robustus archistriatalis are, respectively, 99% and 76% larger in the spring (when the male canaries are producing stable adult song) than in the fall (after the molt and several months of not singing).

Nottebohm's findings support Greenough and Green's (1981) depiction of the nature of plasticity in the adult brain. As summarized by Marx (1982b), Nottebohm's results suggest that

the learning of some motor skills in adulthood depends on the formation of completely new synapses. . . not just modulation of the activities of a fixed set of preexisting synapses. Moreover. . . the formation of neurons may not be limited to very early life, as is generally thought, but may also occur in mature birds. (P. 1125)

Similarly, Cowan (1979, p. 113), in a discussion of the state of knowledge about the development of the brain, indicates that while after "a great deal of research effort it is still not possible to give a complete account of the development of any part of the brain, let alone of the brain as a whole," it nevertheless seems clear that neurons and their development are considerably more complex than had been thought before recent years. To a great extent, this complexity pertains to the plasticity that seems to be evident in the development of neuronal structure and of neurotransmission. For example, "one of the most striking features on the development of neurons is. . . their adoption of a particular mode of transmission (either action potentials or decremental transmission) and the selection of one of two modes of interaction with other cells – either by the formation of conventional synapses, providing for the release of chemical transmitters, or by the formation of gap junctions, providing for electrical interaction among cells" (Cowan, 1979, p. 129). Adding to this complexity is the fact that in some neurons there is a shift from one chemical transmitter (norepinephrine) to another (acetylcholine) when particular environmental conditions are present, and in still other neurons there is a change in the principle ion (from calcium to sodium) used for nerve impulse propagation (Cowan, 1979).

Although such variability describes an instance of neuronal plasticity, there are no clear explanations of these changes. Making such explanation difficult is the fact that during the normal development of the brain, the form of most neurons is modified by an assortment of local mechanical influences that are often nonnormative in timing or character (Cowan, 1979). This responsiveness further underscores the plasticity of neurons and highlights the role of contextual influences – here of a more proximal sort – on neuronal structure and function. For example, the number and distribution of inputs that a neuron receives may affect its final shape.

Age differences in plasticity

Although there is substantial evidence for at least some plasticity in adult animals, of a sort qualitatively similar to that found in early life, certain aspects of plasticity nevertheless seem to be age-related. Thus Greenough and Green (1981, p. 172) acknowledge that the relative sensitivity of the developing neuronal system to extrinsic stimulation may be depicted in terms of critical or sensitive periods, perhaps caused by natural variations in hormones or neurotransmitters (see, e.g., Kasamatsu & Pettigrew, 1979; Lauder & Krebs, 1978), and that the effects of differential experience may be greater during the earlier periods of life.

For example, the sensitivity of several areas of the brain appears to be age-dependent. Fiala, Joyce, and Greenough (1978) found certain effects on the hippocampal granule cell dendrites of rats placed into complex environments, but not of rats in isolated environments, when this differential treatment was administered at weaning, whereas the effects were not seen when 145-day-old rats were given the same differential treatment.

Thus, although adult animals show relatively broad behavioral changes as a consequence of an enriched environment experience, the effects are narrower than those observed when animals are placed in such settings after weaning (Rosenzweig et al., 1972b). Studies by Krech, Rosenzweig, Bennett, and Diamond (Krech, Rosenzweig, & Bennett, 1963; Globus, Rosenzweig, Bennett, & Diamond, 1973; Rosenzweig, Bennett, & Diamond, 1972a,b) on the plasticity of neuronal structures – that is, their responsiveness to contextual influences – indicate that raising young rats in stimulus-enriched versus stimulus-impoverished environments has an effect on brain size, weight, and chemical composition. Rats with stimulus-enriched histories have been found to have larger and heavier brains, greater levels of acetylcholinesterase, more glial cells, and cerebral cortex neurons with more dendritic spines (Globus et al., 1973) than do rats with histories of stimulus impoverishment.

One specific finding has been that the size of certain brain areas, particularly the occipital region of the cerebral cortex (Diamond, 1967), can be influenced by the degree of environmental complexity experienced by an animal. For instance, studies of immature dendrites reveal a loss or lack of development of spines following removal of their normal supply of axonal input (Globus & Scheibel, 1967; Globus, 1975). Similarly, Holloway (1966) found that neurons in the visual cortex of animals reared in enriched environments had more dendritic branching than did those of animals reared in isolation. In addition, studies of sensory deprivation suggest that the activity of the afferent or presynaptic component of the dendrite under study can also influence dendritic morphology (Lynch & Gall, 1979).

Greenough and Green (1981) note that a major instance of age-associated differences in plasticity is the tendency toward net neuronal degeneration in the aged years. Baltes and Baltes (1980) make an analogous point in regard to changes in behavioral plasticity in the aged years. Evidence for continuing flexibility – in intellectual functioning, for example – across the aged years can be reconciled with accompanying decreases in the absolute amount of flexibility (or narrowing of the behavioral "band" within which flexibility can be actualized, Baltes and Baltes argue, by adopting the concept of *selective optimization*, the idea that one may enhance with age an increasingly more circumscribed domain of behaviors. Specifically, Baltes and Baltes address the issue of how to reconcile plasticity in psychological functions across the aged years with biological and, in some cases, psychological decline and vulnerability with aging. They state:

Our tentative view is that biological aging, like psychological aging, is specific (selective) rather than general and that compensation is possible. That such compensatory efforts are effective psychologically is illustrated in our research on plasticity. Yet if aging involves increased biological vulnerability of increasing scope, compensation cannot remedy all dimensions of possible biological vulnerability. Compensation, therefore, becomes increasingly selective. For the time being, we have chosen the term ''selective optimization'' or ''selective efficacy'' (Bandura, 1977) to describe the process in question. (Baltes & Baltes, 1980, p. 59)

Baltes and Baltes (1980) note that selective optimization allows for individualization in the aging years:

If aging individuals show large interindividual differences and remarkable intraindividual plasticity when exposed to supportive (optimizing) environments, one conclusion is that aging is rather idiosyncratic. Life histories would be seen as involving an increasing amount of individualization and specialization....In other words, the developmental pathways and contexts through which individuals travel, with increasing age, show less and less universality and are more and more reflective of individual life experiences. (Baltes & Baltes, 1980, pp. 58-9)

Despite these potential developmental organismic constraints on the quantity of change that may be demonstrable, Greenough and Green (1981) indicate, across-life experience continues to influence brain anatomy. Life events inevitably influence the status of the adult brain and the character of changes associated with aging, a fact that makes possible life-span–oriented preventative or enhancement strategies for intervention. For example, one might target, through historical–ontogenetic strategies, selected areas of functioning within which to encourage selective optimization.

Developmental processes

In Chapter 10 I will return to a discussion of the issues discussed above in terms of intervention. Here it is useful to consider the processes by which experience may influence the brain across development, that is, the processes involved in brain plasticity. In the following section we will consider how processes associated with aging may or may not constrain developmental processes involved in brain plasticity. In the chapter's final section we will consider a major method used in studying processes of brain development – brain transplants – and indicate how this approach may also provide an important tool for intervention.

In their early development most neurons develop more dendritic projections (processes) than are subsequently maintained (Cowan, 1979); all but a few of these processes are retracted over the course of cell maturation. Similarly, developing axons make many more connections than are necessary in the mature cell. Since, according to Cowan (1979, p. 131), the "most important unresolved issue in the development of the brain is the question of how neurons make specific patterns of connections," the fact that many of the early dendritic processes and axon connections are later eliminated raises the key question of what determines a particular connection's survival or loss. Functional facilitation or inhibition seems to be one important factor giving some connections an edge in survival (Cowan, 1979). Thus, particularly in the cortex, neurons are open to a wide array of both intrinsic and environmental influences, and so the study of the brain's ability to reorganize itself in response to external influence is one of the more active, important areas in neurobiological research (Cowan, 1979).

Greenough (1978; see too Changeaux & Danchin, 1977) has advanced the concept of *selective preservation* to describe a process presumed, on the basis of findings of several studies (e.g., Cragg, 1975; Hubel, Wiesel, & Levay, 1977), to be prototypic of normal neuronal development (cf. Purves & Lichtman, 1980). Selective preservation involves the overproduction, in normal neuronal development, of synaptic connections followed by a selective loss of connections; moreover, based on the evidence that use of connections may preserve them from loss, evidence that I noted above was reviewed by Greenough and Green (1981, pp. 161–3), the concept of selective preservation involves the view that those connections that are lost may be ones that are unused or are otherwise inappropriate.

The neuroanatomical concept of selective preservation enhances our understanding of Baltes and Baltes's (1980) behavioral concept of selective optimization, in that the former concept helps explain how experiential history may determine which functions are available for optimization in aging. Indeed, the compatability of Greenough's (1978) and Baltes and Baltes's (1980) concepts suggests the usefulness of research collaboration between neuropsychologists and life-span developmentalists, a collaboration perhaps built on the use of animal models to simulate life-span changes in brain–behavior relations, especially those that may arise in the aged years. Given the impressive amount of evidence in support of Greenough's (1978) concept of selective preservation – evidence derived from data pertinent to the peripheral autonomic nervous system (e.g., Lichtman, 1977) and central nervous system development (e.g., Boothe, Greenough, Lund, & Wrege, 1979) – such collaborative research might be able to account for many (although certainly not all; cf. Greenough & Green, 1981) experience-dependent developmental phenomena of this sort.

Underscoring the potential value of collaboration between neurobehavioral and life-span developmental psychologists is further research by Greenough indicating that the processes involved in these developmental trends relate more "to the processing of information *per se*, rather than to some more generalized (e.g., hormonal, metabolic) effect of experience" (Greenough & Green, 1981, p. 176). Greenough et al. (1979) socially reared littermate pairs of rats for the first 80 days of their lives, after which they were assigned to one or two conditions. A training condition involved 25 days of problem-solving training on the Hebb-Williams (1946) maze, with a new problem being presented each day. In the other condition, rats were merely removed from their cages several times a day. Examination of dendrite branching in pyramidal cells of the occipital cortex after training days revealed marked structural differences between the dendrites of the trained and the nontrained animals. Greenough et al. (1979) are cautious in the interpretation of their results, noting that "any training experience contains various elements (e.g., stress, sensory stimulation, motor activity, etc.) which are not duplicated by the control procedures and which individually or collectively might affect the anatomy of the brain" (p. 296). Nevertheless, consistent with the idea that information processing may be involved in developmental changes in anatomical plasticity at the neuronal level, they point out that their "results are compatible with the notion that anatomical change might underlie some aspect of the memory storage process" (Greenough et al., 1979, p. 296). Indeed, additional maze training studies conducted in Greenough's laboratory (Chang & Greenough, 1978, 1982) suggest that "the changes seen in the brain after training really are associated with the processing of information from the training experience" (Greenough & Green, 1981, pp. 177–8).

In summary, selective preservation processes appear to be among the salient features of neuroanatomical change across life, and the particular connections that are preserved are related to the use made of them across time. Given that experiences involving or promoting information processing may be among those that are associated with the loss or retention of particular connections, it may be that different life histories, involving different opportunities for differential experiences with problem solving, information processing, and so on, result in interindividual differences in connections that are preserved across life; such developmental process – involving critically the link between the organism and its context – may provide the bases of which behavioral functions may be selectively optimized among aged adults. Given this conjecture, it is appropriate to turn now to a consideration of aging and brain plasticity.

Aging and brain plasticity

From the evidence cited so far in this chapter it is possible to conclude that the brain possesses plasticity through adulthood. Moreover, research with animals suggests that minimal cortex may be needed for an organism to engage in substantial and adaptive components of its behavioral repertoire. Murphy, MacLean, and Hamilton (1981) deprived newborn hamsters of their neocortex. Nevertheless, the animals developed normally and displayed the usual hamster-typical behavior patterns – that is, in respect to play and maternal behaviors. However, when the midline limbic convolutions (cingulate and underlying dorsal hippocampal) were also destroyed, deficits arose in these behavior patterns (Murphy et al., 1981). The authors conclude that the latter structures are sufficient, in the absence of neocortex, to enable expression of a wide array of behavior in hamsters.

On the basis of this research and all of the foregoing, we may conclude that there does *not* appear to be a time in the normal life span of studied mammals when flexibility on neural structure can be shown to be completely absent (Green & Greenough, 1981; Lynch & Gerling, 1981). Yet there does appear to be a progressive decrease in the absolute level of malleability as the organism ages. Thus, it is necessary to discuss both features of plasticity that exist in the aged years and the constraints on plasticity associated with aging.

First, Cotman and Nieto-Sampedro (1982) note that time and experience result in an increase in nerve circuit complexity. For instance, neurons of the para-hippocampal gyrus of normal aged humans show marked increases in size and complexity when compared to those of young human adults (Buell & Coleman, 1979).

Results like these indicate that the capacity for growth and change in the CNS is not restricted to the period of early development but instead is retained well into adulthood (Lynch & Gerling, 1981, p. 216); changes in the aging human brain circumscribe only the extent to which growth and change may be expected. Greenough and Green (1981, p. 182) note:

Perhaps the most obvious change in the human brain that occurs with advancing age is a decrease in overall weight. Reduction in weight occurs progressively, with losses in the range of 10–20% between the age of 20 and 90.... This weight reduction occurs regardless of brain pathology although it appears to be less severe in healthy subjects.

Greenough and Green note that although neuron loss is variable, occurring at different rates in different areas of the brain and for different types of cells, neuron death may be the major reason for this weight loss. Moreover, they imply that with brain pathology the weight loss may be more severe. Findings by Whitehouse et al. (1982) support such an inference. These investigators found that neurons of the nucleus basalis of Meynert, a distinct population of basal forebrain neurons, undergo a profound (greater than 75%) and selective degeneration in the brains of patients with Alzheimer's disease and with senile dementia of the Alzheimer's type. It should be here noted – because of its relevance to our discussion of neurotransmitters in Chapter 5 – that the nucleus basalis of

Meynert is a major source of cholinergic innervation of the cerebral cortex, and the demonstration by Whitehouse et al. (1982) of selective degeneration of such neurons represents the first documentation of a loss of a transmitter-specific neuronal population in a major disorder of higher cortical function.

Greenough and Green (1981) believe, however, that perhaps more important than neuron death in accounting for changes in brain–behavior relations in aging are losses in neuronal connections, losses that have been reported often in the aged, especially in pathological cases. For instance, although the young adults studied by Buell and Coleman (1979) had, as noted, less complex dendritic trees in the parahippocampal gyrus than did nonpathological aged adults, the young adults had more extensive dendritic trees than did demented aged adults. Methodological and other problems (see Bondareff, 1981) have served to limit the studies of changes during aging in synaptic numbers, however, and the results of the few studies are not decisive in indicating the extent to which synapse loss per se is a general feature of aging brains. Thus, Bondareff (1981, p. 143) states:

Loss of synapses will, of course, result from a loss of neurons and it is a long-taught maxim of neuropathology that the number of neurons declines with age. This decline, which is reflected by the general pessimism of agism...is not ubiquitous and in some cases not even certain.

For example, in a study comparing the brains of normal people aged 65 to 89 with the brains of mentally deficient and neurosurgical patients, Cragg (1975) found a loss of neither synapses nor neurons in the cerebral cortex of either group. In a study comparing 3-month-old with 24-month-old rats, however, fewer synapses in dentate gyrus granule cells were found in the older rats (Bondareff & Geinisman, 1976; Geinisman & Bondareff, 1976; Glick & Bondareff, 1979), although the loss of synapses appeared to depend primarily on changes in the presynaptic (as opposed to postsynaptic) neuron (Bondareff, 1981).

Thus, whether synapse loss is seen in aging may depend on the area of the brain and the type of cell being studied. Nevertheless, the capacity of neurons to regenerate lost connections does appear to decline with age. For instance, Bregman and Goldberger (1982) found that although spinal cord damage in neonatal cats has different effects on different spinal pathways, corticospinal projections exhibit anatomical plasticity – forming an aberrant pathway that bypasses the lesion – whereas brain stem–spinal pathways undergo massive retrograde degeneration. However, neither of these two types of change occurs in adult cats. In addition, in cats operated on as neonates motor function is spared, but this is not the case in cats operated on as adults. In turn, Scheff, Bernardo, and Cotman (1978) found that adrenergic neurons in the senescent rat retain some capacity to sprout following deafferentation of the septal area and dentate gyrus, but only at diminished levels. Similarly, Cotman and Scheff (1979) found that the extent and rate with which commisural and associational projections sprouted, after lesions were made in the entorhinal cortex of young and of aged rats, were significantly less in the older group.

Lynch and Gerling (1981) believe that researchers are close to identifying the mechanism by which this age-associated decrement in axonal plasticity occurs; for instance, they believe that gradual changes in the astrocyte population over the life of an animal may inhibit axonal growth (cf. Selkoe, Ihara, & Salazar, 1982). Positive identification of such a mechanism promises to open the path to experimental manipulation and ultimately to intervention.

Among other investigators seeking to uncover the mechanisms involved in age changes in plasticity and to provide information potentially applicable to intervention (e.g., see Enna, Samorajski, & Beer, 1981; Holliday, Huschtscha, & Kirkwood, 1981), Levin, Janda, Joseph, Ingram, and Roth (1981) note that with increasing age there is often an impaired ability to respond and adapt to various stimuli, such as drugs, hormones, neurotransmitters, and physical and chemical agents. Their research has documented that some of the mechanisms involved in these response changes involve alterations in receptors, in cell membranes, in nuclei, and in cyclic neucleotide metabolism. Much research has been devoted to attempting to retard the aging process and its associated decrements. However, the only confirmed method of life-span extension in mammals at this writing involves dietary manipulation (Levin et al., 1981). Levin et al. believe that such intervention may act by modifying disease patterns and thus the associated impairment of physiological systems. However, researchers still do not know the actual mechanism by which dietary intervention extends the mammalian life span, and Levin et al. note that little research has been devoted to assessing the relation between dietary manipulation and the functional manifestations of senescence. Focusing on the degeneration and reduced responsiveness of the striatal dopaminergic system, one of the best-documented instances of functional impairment of the aging mammalian brain, Levin et al. (1981) appraised the effects of dietary restriction on normative age-related loss of receptors for dopamine (a neurotransmitter to be discussed in the next chapter) from the rat corpus striatum.

Levin et al. (1981) subjected male rats to dietary restriction by feeding and fasting them on alternate days. This intervention substantially retarded the normal age-associated loss of striatal dopamine receptors in the brain. More interestingly, the mean survival time of the rats on this restricted diet was increased by approximately 40% over control rats given free access to food. Most interestingly, dopamine receptor concentrations in the striata of 24-month-old rats that had been on a restricted diet since weaning were 50% higher than those of similarly aged control rats – essentially the same as in 3- to 6-month-old control rats.

Thus, the brain's structures (here dopamine receptors) are available targets of intervention (here of a dietary nature). The research by Levin et al. suggests not only that such intervention may extend the life spans of target organisms, but also that the brains of these organisms may not age as fast as nontreated organisms. Thus, the treated organisms not only live longer, but in a sense stay "younger" as they grow older.

Returning to the research of Nottebohm and his colleagues, we may note findings that also serve to suggest means to intervene – here in respect to hormonal administration – in the potential mechanisms of aging. DeVoogd and Nottebohm (1981) found that gonadal hormones induce dendritic growth in the adult avian (canary) brain and, more interestingly, can significantly alter sex-linked functions associated with brain structures. For example, singing, typical only of males, was exhibited by ovariectomized adult female canaries treated with physiological doses of testosterone. Other, nonmale gonadal hormones (dihydrotestosterone and estradiol) did not have this effect. In addition, in the testosterone-treated female birds the neurons of the nucleus robustus archistrialalis, a forebrain nucleus for song control, exhibited dendritic trees resembling those of intact males; however, the corresponding neurons of the birds treated with other hormones exhibited dendrites that resembled those of intact females. Nevertheless, despite the specific effects associated with the testosterone treatment, *all* hormone-treated groups exhibited dendrites significantly longer than those of the untreated ovariectomized females. Thus, from this evidence one may conclude that a general influence of gonadal hormones is to induce dendritic growth in the adult avian brain (DeVoogd & Nottebohm, 1981).

Despite the promise these studies hold for understanding and manipulating presumed mechanisms of aging, the current status of the literature does not contradict the normative appropriateness of Bondareff's (1981) conclusion that "if the distribution of synapses continually changes during life, that is, if synapses are continually being formed, destroyed and reformed, then the formative process must fail in senescence" (p. 146).

Thus, insofar as plasticity, while present across life, is, with increasing age, applicable to a possibly smaller number of constituent "units" (e.g., neurons, synapses) and to a possibly narrower range of functions (e.g., cognitive or behavioral attributes), Greenough's (1978) concept of "selective preservation" seems appropriate for depicting key neuroanatomical changes that are part of this age-associated change in plasticity. Similarly appropriate is Baltes and Baltes's (1980) notion of "selective optimization" for describing the extent to which one may capitalize on the aging organism's diminished, but still present, capability for flexibility.

The issue of optimization returns us to the topic of intervention. It will be useful to conclude this chapter with a discussion of how the use of one of the major methodologies that has been employed to study processes of brain development has led, more recently, to providing avenues for capitalizing on brain plasticity and for intervening to enhance human life.

The use of transplants in the study of brain development and in intervention

For many years neuroscientists have been able to successfully transplant neural tissue of amphibians, fish, and birds into conspecifics. In recent years similar techniques have been used with mammalian brains after it was found that "mammalian brain tissue would not only survive transplantation to a new location but would develop normally" (Marx, 1982c, p. 340); this demonstration has provided evidence to counter the "belief that mammalian brains, unlike those of amphibians and fish, would have little recuperative power if they were damaged as they would be during transplant surgery" (Marx, 1982c, p. 340).

Being able to transplant tissue successfully into the mammalian brain gives one the ability to experimentally test hypotheses about variables in brain development (e.g., pertaining to the position or to the timing of contributions of particular neuronal tissue). Several studies indicate that transplanted brain tissue makes and receives connections from other brain areas (e.g., Arendash & Gorski, 1982) and that these connections are often the appropriate ones.

However, as with age-related constraints on plasticity, there are age-related constraints on the success of transplantation. Although investigators such as Arendash and Gorski (1982) have transplanted neonatal brain tissue (from the preoptic area of male rat neonates into the preoptic area of female littermates) with positive results (the females showed increased masculine and feminine sexual behavior during adulthood, thereby suggesting that functional connections developed between the transplanted neural tissue and the host brain), most researchers believe that fetal tissue is best to use in transplantation work. This belief is based on the fact that neural tissues taken even during the perinatal period have not been successfully transplanted as often as have tissues taken duing the fetal period and on the observation of what may be an age-associated advantage of fetal neural cells to divide more readily than the neural cells of neonates or still older organisms (Marx, 1982c).

Another age-related consideration that seems to exist among many researchers in this area involves the fact that fetal tissue is usually transplanted into neonates; again, this procedural preference is a result of the presumably greater growth and regenerative capacities of neonatal as compared with adult brain tissue (cf. Marx, 1982c). Nevertheless, we have seen in this chapter considerable evidence for the continued plasticity of both the adult and the aged brain. Indeed, both basic research and intervention with both animal and human adults have been found to be quite encouraging.

Nieto-Sampedro, Lewis, Cotman, Manthorpe, Skaper, Barbin, Longo, and Varon (1982) made a cavity in the brain (entorhinal cortex) of developing and adult rats, and inserted a small piece of absorbent gel into the cavity to collect fluid secreted into the wound. As the authors note, the potential of CNS tissue to recover from injury depends on the substances and processes that support neuron survival (neuronotrophic factors); thus they assayed the fluid that was secreted into the wound with sympathetic and parasympathetic neurons in culture to determine neuronotrophic activity. The authors found that the wounds in the brains of both the developing and the adult rats comparably stimulated the accumulation of neuronotrophic factors and that the activity of these factors increased over the first few days after infliction of the damage.

The importance of this study for the present discussion is its suggestion that the adult mammalian brain retains – at a level comparable to that of the developing brain – the processes needed to recover from injury – for example as would occur if a transplant operation were conducted. Thus, if one were to try to intervene with transplantation to correct brain damage of some sort, the recuperative ability of the adult brain would be sufficient to justify the intervention. Indeed, just such interventions have been successful with both rats and monkeys. In 1982 work with humans began (Kolata, 1982; *New York Times*, July 25, 1982, sec. A, p. 15).

In the summer of 1982 in Karolinska Hospital in Stockholm a man seriously affected by Parkinson's disease became the first human known to have tissue transplanted into his brain. The movement disorders that mark Parkinsonianism are associated with a decrement in the production of a neurotransmitter – dopamine (to be discussed in greater detail in Chapter 5) – produced in the brain in the substantia nigra. The surgeons capitalized on the fact that transplants directly into the brain bypass the blood–brain barrier – a barrier that keeps numerous dangerous substances from reaching the brain but also restricts the passage of immunological cells into the brain that would "attack" the foreign (i.e., transplanted) material. The surgeons transplanted adrenal gland tissue directly into the caudate nucleus of the brain. Adrenal gland tissue was used because the adrenal medulla makes dopamine as a minor product; it was hoped this tissue would grow and produce dopamine (Kolata, 1982).

One of the neurosurgeons on the project, Lars Olson, concluded that the procedure proved somewhat successful. He noted that when the patient awoke, the attending scientists saw "no immediate or dramatic symptoms.... If anything, he was somewhat better.... There was a slight improvement, but nothing sensational" (quoted in Kolata, 1982, p. 342). For instance the patient required less medication, only 80–85% of the levels he previously needed (Kokata, 1982).

While this clinical intervention does not have the features of a controlled experiment (e.g., there was no sham control group), and indeed while such an experiment would be unethical at this time, the results of this clinical intervention are not discouraging. In fact, these results combined with the positive results that have been derived from animal experimentation form a good basis for being encouraged about the possibility of using brain transplants in the future to correct human brain–behavior problems. Indeed, some researchers predict that "brain transplants will be clinically feasible in this country within five to 10 years" (Kolata, 1982, p. 342).

Insofar as the animal work is concerned, much of it has capitalized on the link between the hippocampus and memory functions, noted earlier in this chapter. For example, after a group of Swedish and British researchers (Björklund, Stenevi, Lund, Iversen, & Dunnett) produced lesions in rats' hippocampus, the rats' short-term memory was lost (Kolata, 1982). When fetal cells that produce various neurotransmitters (e.g., acetylcholine – also discussed in greater detail in Chapter 5) were transplanted into the hippocampus, the rats' memories were restored – for example, they were able to learn T-mazes (Kolata, 1982). Similarly, when Perlow, Freed, Hoffer, Seiger, Olson, and Wyatt (1979) transplanted fetal dopamine neurons into rats' brains, they found a reduction of the motor abnormalities resulting from lesions of the substantia nigra. Other evidence of the success of transplantation comes from the research of Gash, Sladek, and Sladek (1980), who report that vasopressin neurons, transplanted from normal rat fetuses into the third ventricle of adult rats, alleviated the polydipsia and polyuria of the hosts. These findings suggest that symptoms resulting from a congenital defect in the central nervous system of an adult mammal can be ameliorated by transplanted neurons, and they underscore the idea that even in adults there is considerable potential nervous system plasticity.

In sum, not only does the brain retain at least some capacity for growth and change across life, but it also maintains a capacity for self-repair across this time span; and because it is an "immunologically privileged site" (Kolata, 1982), the brain may remain available across adulthood to be a target of interventions aimed at correcting through tissue transplantation major defects in structure and/or brain–behavior relations.

Conclusions

On the basis of both evolutionary and ontogenetic evidence, the character of the neuroanatomy of the human brain is such as to provide a key basis of human plasticity. Not only does such plasticity, which exists among developing, mature, and even aging neural structures, enable humans to respond to changes in their physical and social context; but in turn, changes in the physical and, perhaps especially, the social context appear to provide a key basis for neuroanatomical development, change, and hence plasticity. Thus, this link between physical and social experience provides a key basis for stressing the importance of multidisciplinary research and intervention. As we turn now to another key basis of human plasticity – the nature of human neurochemistry and the role of neurotransmitters – we will again see numerous reasons for taking a multidisciplinary approach to research and intervention.

5 Human neurochemistry and the role of neurotransmitters

In many ways neurons are like other living cells – for example, they can generate energy and repair and maintain themselves. However, neurons have unique functions not shared with other cells. Among these specialized features is the transmission of nerve impulses and those processes associated with the ability of neurons to produce and release neurotransmitters (Iversen, 1979). More than anything else in the human brain, its neurochemical characteristics provide unequivocal evidence for the plasticity of the human organism.

According to Thompson (1981), the key to understanding the actual character of human plasticity provided by the brain lies in an understanding of the chemical synapse and thus neurotransmitters. In the human brain most of the synaptic connections among neurons are chemical. As opposed to electrical synapses, which are common in many invertebrates and which work like an electrical transformer – that is, output is determined by input and is unmodifiable – chemical synapses are very plastic (Thompson, 1981). There are over 30 different known or suspected brain transmitters; each has a characteristic excitatory or inhibitory effect on neurons (Iversen, 1979). In addition, neurotransmitters are localized in specific brain regions.

Due to advances in techniques that allow for the selective staining of neurons containing a particular transmitter, thus facilitating the study of the functional chemistry of the brain, researchers have been able to map the anatomical distribution of individual transmitters in specific neuronal pathways (Iversen, 1979). For example, the monoamines norepinephrine, dopamine, and serotonin are the best-mapped neurotransmitters. Each has been found to be involved in important biological and behavioral functions. As we will see below, these links provide bases for behavioral intervention. In addition, monoamines as well as other neurotransmitters either resemble the normal constituents of certain foods, particularly amino acids from proteins, or, like dopamine, are manufactured in the brain from an amino acid found in the normal American diet (Thompson, 1981). Moreover, other nutrients, such as calcium, seem to be implicated as moderators of neurotransmitter action (Thompson, 1981). Thus, because nutritional intake and dietary habits may impact on neurotransmitter presence and level, modification of diet and/or eating behavior may provide a means for usefully altering brain chemistry (Wurtman, 1982). Successful instances of such multilevel intervention efforts exist.

Altering neurotransmitters through nutritional intervention

Wurtman (1982) notes that in some important ways nutrients act like drugs that alter neurotransmission. He states:

A nutrient is a food substance that in most cases supplies either the energy or the molecular building blocks the body requires. A drug is a substance given for its effect on a specific organ or type of cell. Whereas all healthy people need essentially the same nutrients, a drug would ordinarily be recommended only for people with a particular disease or condition.... three nutrients,... when they are administered in the pure form or simply ingested in food, can act like drugs. They give rise to important changes in the chemical composition of structures in the brain. The changes can modify brain function, particularly in people with certain metabolic or neurologic diseases.

Two of the nutrients are the amino acids tryptophan and tyrosine. Amino acids are the building blocks of proteins, and so tryptophan and tyrosine are present in most foods. The third nutrient is choline, a component of lecithin; egg yolks, liver and soybeans are notably rich in lecithin. The composition and function of the brain can be altered by tryptophan, tyrosine and choline because they are the precursors of neurotransmitters.... Tryptophan is converted in the terminals of certain neurons into the neurotransmitter serotonin. In other cells choline is converted into the transmitter acetylcholine. In still another population of cells tyrosine serves as the precursor of dopamine, norepinephrine and epinephrine, which are collectively called the catecholamine transmitters. An increase in the brain level of a precursor enhances the synthesis of the corresponding neurotransmitter product. The enhanced synthesis can in turn cause the neuron to release more transmitter molecules when it fires, amplifying the transmission of signals from the neuron to the cells it innervates. (Wurtman, 1982, p. 50)

Given the link between dietary intake of neurotransmitter precursors and nervous system activity, it may be important to gain knowledge of the social and psychological processes involved in eating habits and the familial, intergenerational, cultural, and ecological variables affecting the presence or absence of particular foods in the diet in order to fully understand the individual and/or group presence of various neurotransmitter precursors and other supportive chemicals. Indeed, several conference papers and books have recently been devoted to the study of the use of dietary precursors to control neurotransmitter synthesis.

For example, Barbeau, Growdon, and Wurtman (1979) present evidence for the use of choline and lecithin in this regard. Their data indicate that administration of these dietary precursors of acetylcholine can ameliorate behavioral and psychological disorders – for example, tardive dyskinesia, memory disorders, and psychoaffective disorders such as mania.

In this regard Wurtman (1982, p. 50) has noted that choline and tyrosine can "amplify neurotransmission selectively, increasing it at some synapses but not at others. It may be possible to exploit such selectivity to develop novel therapeutic agents for several diseases, including hypertension, some forms of depression, Parkinsonism and some memory disorders of old people."

To illustrate this potential interventive use, consider tardive dyskinesia, a disorder marked by uncontrollable movements of the face and upper body and often caused by repeated administration of antipsychotic drugs. A treatment that at least temporarily ameliorates the disordered movement is administration of physostignine, a drug that increases the levels of acetylcholine in the brain by blocking its degredation by cholinesterase. Similar therapeutic success can also be achieved by increasing brain acetylcholine through administering choline (Wurtman, 1982).

Another key outcome of the work of Wurtman and his associates at the Massachusetts Institute of Technology that has important implications for intervention is their determination of how dietarily introduced tryptophan passes through the blood–brain barrier to influence serotonin synthesis (Kolata, 1976). This feature of Wurtman's work is especially important for the development of dietary intervention tools because a major limitation faced by all researchers seeking to influence brain function via ingested or injected chemicals is the existence of the blood–brain barrier – that is, as noted in Chapter 4, that feature of brain structure and function precluding various exogenous (and even some endogenous) chemicals from passing from the bloodstream into the brain's cells. By determining how tryptophan is transported through this barrier, the Wurtman group have overcome a major obstacle facing interventionists interested in changing brain and behavior through the introduction of "foreign" materials into the body and have provided hope that other instances may be forthcoming (as we have indeed seen they are, at the level of molecular biology, with advances in recombinant DNA technology). For example, in the case of serotonin – a neurotransmitter that has been linked to avoidance learning, the effects of hallucinogenic drugs, sleep, pain sensitivity, control of eating, and pituitary hormone release – dietary intervention effective in influencing brain synthesis of serotonin has obvious potential use in numerous areas of behavioral and physiological functioning.

Other lines of evidence also suggest the usefulness of dietarily administered neurotransmitter precursors as intervention strategies. Harrell, Capp, David, Peerless, and Ravitz (1981), for example, explored the hypothesis that mental retardations are in part conditions whose amelioration requires an augmented supply of one or more nutrients. The authors studied 16 school-age retarded children whose initial IQs ranged from below 20 to 70 and who were given a nutritional supplement or placebo during an 8-month period. The supplement contained 8 minerals in moderate amounts and 11 vitamins, mostly in relatively large amounts. The 5 children who received supplements increased their IQs by 5 to 10 points, whereas the 11 subjects given placebos showed virtually no change; the difference between the two groups was statistically significant. Moreover, when the subjects who had initially received placebos were then given the supplements, an increase of at least 10 IQ points per subject was seen. In addition, 3 of 5 subjects who were given supplements across the 8-month period showed even greater IQ gains, and 3 of 4 children with Down's syndrome gained between 10 and 25 IQ points and also showed some physical changes toward normal.

While the data of Harrell et al. (1981) can only be considered preliminary in nature, they do coincide with those reported by other investigations; and although the authors claim no direct links between the dietary supplements they provided and neurotransmitter synthesis, a major implication of their work, especially in light of information provided by Wurtman (1982) and by Barbeau et al. (1979), is that dietary interventions may be useful for ameliorating or preventing cognitive and behavioral problems arising from disorders in normative neurotransmitter production.

Indeed, several lines of evidence converge to suggest the plausability of this inference. Winick (1980) notes that malnutrition early in life can cause developmental abnormalities in the brain, and that the earlier malnutrition begins, the "greater the potential for interfering with cell division and ultimately reducing the number of brain cells" (p. 6). Studies he conducted with rats demonstrate that early malnutrition causes a reduction in the concentration of n-acetylneurominic acid (NANA), a chemical secretion of neurons that appears to facilitate nerve impulse transmission in the tips of dendrites.

Winick points out, however, that the deficits of early malnutrition can be reversed. As may be expected, an intervention composed of proper nutrition can lead to reversal. However, other environmental "enrichments" can also be used to correct the deficits produced by malnutrition. For example, indicative of the responsivity of brain chemistry to contextual influence, and thus illustrative of the potential use of collaborative research among behavioral, social, and neuroscientists, is the finding that environmental stimulation increases the concentration of NANA. Morgan and Winick (1980), for instance, manipulated the nutritional and early stimulation conditions of rat pups during the first 3 weeks of life. Early stimulation reduced the effects of malnutrition on activity in an open-field test at 21 days of life, and the improved behavioral performance was associated with significantly higher NANA content in the brain. Moreover, at a retest conducted at age 6 months, the rats receiving the early stimulation performed better on a maze-learning task and again had higher brain levels of NANA. In addition, "injection of NANA into malnourished animals increases its concentration at the synapses of the dendrites and prevents the expected behavioral abnormalities" (Winick, 1980, p. 13).

Conclusions. We may summarize the above research by noting that diet, brain chemicals, and environmental stimulation, as can be introduced, for example, by cognitive–behavioral or social interventions, appear to exist in a system of reciprocal relations; diet affects brain chemicals and behavior; context and behavior affects brain chemicals; brain chemicals affect behavior. While we will have more to say about the alteration of brain chemicals and of cognitive–behavioral and social interventions as means to enhance human functioning, two points should be emphasized here.

First, the research of Winick (1980), as well as that of others from independent laboratories (e.g., McKay, Sinisterra, McKay, Gomez, & Lloreda, 1978), suggests that nutritional interventions, especially when combined with environmental stimulation changes – for example, in regard to type of social interaction (Morgan & Winick, 1980) or family constitution (Winick, Jaroslow, & Winer, 1978) – can be effective means of changing behavior and brain structure, composition, and function. Second, such plasticity underscores – in the area of nutritional intervention and brain structure and function – the point made by Brim and Kagan (1980): Evidence from numerous disciplines indicates that early features of development do not necessarily completely constrain those of later life; rather, the organism remains open to influence, its processes remain plastic, and it retains its flexibility. Indeed, as Winick (1980, p. 13) notes, "In the past thirty years we have come full circle. Whereas initially we believed that early malnutrition invariably led to structural and chemical changes in the brain that, in turn, left permanent behavioral scars, the current data suggest that... the changes are potentially reversible."

That nutritional interventions may be effective means to alter brain chemistry, and thus behavior, is more than a tentative conclusion. It is, at this writing, a well-replicated observation. Dietary interventions are of use in influencing both normal and disordered behavioral and physiological functioning linked to various neurotransmitters, and there are indeed quite well-known illustrations of this point. Scriver and Clow (1980a, b) cite phenylketonuria (PKU) as a classic example of the workings of human biochemistry/genetics inasmuch as (1) it is a genetic disorder that is inherited as an autosomal-recessive trait according to Mendel's law of segregation; (2) it is an "inborn" error of metabolism, and thus illustrates a key principle of gene action – genetic factors specify chemical reactions and human biochemical individuality; and, most importantly, (3) it is a disease that occurs only when the mutant allele is expressed in a specific environment, one containing an abundance of the essential amino acid L-phenylalanine. Thus, PKU well illustrates the contextual interactions I have been emphasizing. Moreover, it is an excellent example in the context of the present discussion of the use of dietary intervention because it is possible to predict and prevent the genetic and social effects of PKU (e.g., mental retardation and the social stigma associated with being either retarded or the parents of a retarded child); such intervention can be achieved because PKU causes mental retardation only in environments with the normal levels of dietary phenylalanine, and to treat (prevent) PKU's effects, one need only control the patient's exposure to dietary phenylalanine (Scriver & Clow, 1980a, b).

Diet, neurotransmitters, and behavior: bidirectional relations

A major point in the above discussion is that given known and potential links between neurotransmitters, other brain chemicals, dietary precursors of these substances, and behavior, it would be important for scientists to know the psychological, social, and cultural variables that lead individuals and groups to adopt or fail to adopt diets with necessary levels of particular precursors; in addition, behavioral and cognitive–behavioral interventions (e.g., Kendall & Hollon, 1979) would be useful for facilitating adoption of desirable dietary habits. Here again is the need for a multidisciplinary effort in research and intervention. The links between neurotransmitters and dietary/eating habits make clear a bidirectional relation between neurochemistry and behavior: Neurotransmitters affect one's behavioral and psychological functioning, and dietary habits and eating behavior may affect the ingestion of appropriate neurotransmitter precursors and thus the presence of the neurotransmitters themselves.

To further illustrate this bidirectionality, eating behavior appears to be related to the function of several neurotransmitters, including the monoamines. In particular, levels of the peptide neurotransmitter beta-endorphin (which will be discussed in greater detail below) have been found to be influenced by levels of food ingestion (Krieger & Martin, 1981b). Gambert, Garthwaite, Pontzer, and Hagen (1980) report a decline in hypothalamic beta-endorphin among rats that were fasted for two to three days, and Einhorn, Young, and Landsberg (1982) found that among spontaneously hypertensive rats fasting lowered blood pressure to an extent greater than in normotensive rats, and further found that this hypotensive effect of fasting was mediated by beta-endorphin.

In turn, research by Mandenoff, Fumeron, Apfelbaum, and Margules (1982) links increased beta-endorphin production and overeating. These authors note that increasing the palatability of food has two, opposing effects: It promotes overeating, and it promotes higher caloric output; that is, energy is expended by the behavior of eating per se. Of course, the expenditure of energy in the act of eating is not sufficient to compensate for overeating, and as a consequence obesity may result. The authors, studying such diet-induced obesity in rats, administered the drug naloxone, which blocks the action of beta-endorphin. We will have reason to discuss again the use of naloxone in studies assessing the possible effects of endorphins on behavior. Here, suffice it to say that repeated administration of naloxone completely abolished this type of obesity. The drug had this effect by both reducing overeating and by increasing energy expenditure, suggesting that endorphins "encourage obesity in two ways – by stimulating appetite for palatable foods and by reducing energy expenditures" (Mandenoff et al., 1982, p. 1536).

Of course, the etiology of obesity studied by Mandenoff et al. (1982) is not the only known one, and similarly, beta-endorphin is not the only neurotransmitter that has been linked to obesity. For example, the body weights of genetically obese rats can be greatly reduced by long-term ingestion of L-dopa, the substance from which dopamine is manufactured in the brain (Hemmes, Pack, & Hirsch, 1979).

In sum, if the results linking neurotransmitters to overeating and obesity were found to be applicable to humans, appropriate intervention might involve more than just precursor administration. In addition, social and behavioral interventions might be warranted. For example, in a case where family history variables indicated that obesity was influenced by intergenerational transmissions, family counseling or social network changes might be useful. In turn, if inappropriate eating habits were evident in an age group wherein it was difficult to assure compliance with drug therapy (e.g., in adolescence), behavioral and/or cognitive–behavioral interventions would be helpful. However, before such multidisciplinary approaches to intervention may proceed with any general expectation of success, several major problems associated with the interventive use of dietary precursors of neurotransmitters need to be solved.

Current limitations in the use of dietary precursors as intervention tools

Wurtman (1982) has provided a useful view of the state of affairs regarding the use of dietary precursors of neurotransmitters for treating disease. Writing about the known link between lecithin administration and cholinergic neurotransmission, he indicates that although "any disease state known to result from inadequate cholinergic neurotransmission, in any part of the body, now becomes a candidate for treatment with lecithin given either alone or as an adjunct to drug therapy," with the exception of tardive dyskinesia "too little information is available to sustain even tentative conclusions as to lecithin's therapeutic efficacy" (p. 57). Wurtman further notes that

The diseases currently generating the most interest as candidates for lecithin therapy are the memory disorders associated with old age. Aging brings with it a loss of neurons in the brain, and cholinergic neurons seem to be particularly vulnerable. The hippocampus, a region of the brain known to be essential for the formation of new memories, has a particularly large number of cholinergic neurons. The administration to young people of drugs such as scopolamine, which block cholinergic transmission, causes short-term memory impairments similar to those observed in the aged. For these reasons it seems possible that treatments calculated to increase brain acetylcholine may be effective in some patients with memory disorders. (p. 57)

Bartus, Dean, Beer, and Lippa (1982) have reviewed evidence pertinent to this "cholinergic hypothesis" of geriatric memory dysfunction. Such evidence includes the facts that (1) significant cholinergic dysfunctions occur in the CNS of the aged and of the demented; (2) relations exist between these cholinergic changes and memory loss; (3) memory deficits similar to those seen in the aged and in the demented can be experimentally induced in young subjects by artificially blocking cholinergic mechanisms; and (4) under specific, highly controlled conditions reliable improvements can be achieved in aged subjects' memories by cholinergic stimulation (Bartus et al. 1982; Enna, Samorajski, & Beer, 1981; Struble, Cork, Whitehouse, & Price, 1982). Despite this evidence, Bartus et al. (1982) suggest that translation of this knowledge into a useful intervention tool may not lie in the immediate future, noting that "conventional attempts to reduce memory impairments in clinical trials have not been therapeutically successful" (p. 408).

Wurtman (1982) describes some of the problems that need to be addressed in order to develop generally useful therapies for these memory dysfunctions. First, there is a need for a clinical basis for classifying memory-impaired patients into subgroups on the basis of the etiology of their problem; for example, Wurtman believes that people now all grouped together on the basis of having senile dementia or Alzheimer's disease will be found eventually to be people with several distinct disorders. Second, Wurtman points to the need for well-validated tests of memory, especially ones sensitive to changes in memory and useful for indexing the person's ecologically representative memory functions. Third, problems associated with preparing doses of lecithin sufficiently pure and sufficiently large to insure an adequate test of a treatment make difficult the validation of a measure of memory.

Thus, formidable problems remain before the research documenting the role of diet and of dietary precursors of neurotransmitters in psychosocial functioning can be translated into generally useful interventions. Nevertheless, the nature of the links between diet, dietary precursors, and behavior, and the nature of the problems that remain to be solved before useful interventions can be established, are all of a multilevel character. They underscore the usefulness of a multidisciplinary approach to research and intervention, as does work being conducted on the role of neurotransmitters themselves in physical and psychosocial functioning and on the use of neurotransmitters themselves in intervention. We consider this research next.

Neurotransmitters: roles in physical and psychosocial functioning and as intervention tools

Not only may we intervene dietarily to alter the presence or level of various neurotransmitters. In addition, as neuroscientists have been increasingly able to identify, isolate, and synthesize neurotransmitters and more and more information is being obtained about the role of neurotransmitters in behavioral functioning and in the development of diseases, scientists have been attempting to use neurotransmitters directly to alter behavior and/or ameliorate disease.

As an example of links between neurotransmitters and behavior, the neurotransmitter norepinephrine, concentrated in the brain stem (in the locus coeruleus), plays a role in the maintenance of arousal, in sleep, and in mood regulation (Iversen, 1979). And regeneration of the neurons concentrated in the substantia nigra (in the midbrain) and containing the monoamine dopamine is associated with the movement problems (e.g., muscular rigidity, tremors) of Parkinson's disease (Iversen, 1979; Thompson, 1981). Moreover, there is evidence to suggest that depression is linked to a decrease in the level of monoamines in the brain. Collis and Shepherd (1980) note that a general conclusion of most researchers studying the behavioral influences of such neurotransmitters is that some, if not all, depressions are associated with either an absolute or relative deficiency of catecholamines, particularly norepinephrine, at functionally important adrenergic receptor sites in the brain.

In addition, Iversen (1979) notes that abnormally high concentrations of dopamine and dopamine receptors have been found in the brains of deceased schizophrenics, in particular in the limbic system, which is involved in emotional behavior. Iversen suggests that dopamine receptors in the limbic system may be a useful target for antipsychotic drugs. Moreover, in addition to its possible role in emotional disorders, dopamine has been linked to diabetes. Lozovsky, Saller, and Kopin (1981) report that the number of dopamine receptors and the pattern of central dopaminergic transmission may be altered in diabetes; for example, receptor binding is increased.

The interventive use of neurotransmitters is already much in evidence, as illustrated by research derived from knowledge of the link between dopamine and Parkinsonism. As noted in Chapter 4, administration of L-dopa reverses the symptoms of Parkinsonism. In Parkinsonism, presumably due to cell death, there is not a sufficient level of dopamine produced to provide for normal movement; L-dopa administration apparently induces remaining cells to increase dopamine production to a level sufficient to reverse the disorder. In addition, Thompson (1981) points out that there may be a similar use for L-dopa in the treatment of movement disorders among the aged that resemble Parkinsonism; he describes recent research conducted with aged rats that indicated that L-dopa administration reverses impaired movement.

The potential importance of neurotransmitters in intervention is not limited to monoamines. Another major example of this potential relates to research with gamma-aminobutyric acid (GABA), an amino acid. GABA is the brain's major inhibitory neurotransmitter that, like dopamine, is manufactured in neurons from an amino acid found in the normal diet. Deficits in brain GABA have been implicated in a variety of disorders; Huntington's chorea, anxiety, and epilepsy are examples. In certain types of epilepsy, for example, neurons that produce GABA are apparently not present; without the inhibition that GABA provides, excitation is not appropriately diminished and an epileptic seizure occurs (Thompson, 1981).

Other neurotransmitters are implicated in the production of epilepsy – that is, considered epileptogenic. A group of neurotransmitters to be discussed in greater detail below is the neuropeptides, and as we will see, many of these neuropeptides, specifically endorphins and enkephalins, have analgesic (pain-relieving) properties. Moreover, some of these neuropeptides also seem to be epileptogenic. For example, while particular levels of enkephalin, when injected at specific brain sites (e.g., the periaqueductal gray matter of the midbrain) causes analgesia without seizures, these same levels cause seizures without analgesia when injected near the dorsomedial nucleus of the thalamus (Krieger & Martin, 1981b).

In sum, although not yet generally feasible, it may be possible one day to prevent, arrest, or ameliorate several diseases and/or their effects through administration of neurotransmitters. Indeed, as we will see below, there is research that suggests the feasibility of intervention with both animals and humans through administration of particular (peptide) neurotransmitters.

Neuropeptides

Neither the monoamines nor GABA have been the neurotransmitters attracting the most recent attention among neurochemists. With the discovery in recent years of a new group of neurochemicals, the *neuropeptides* (molecules containing chains of from 2 to 39 amino acids), particularly endorphins and enkephalins, several new areas of research have opened up.

There are several reasons for the intense interest in the study of peptide neurotransmitters. First, it is estimated that nonpeptide neurotransmitters may account for only 40% of the synapses in the central nervous system (Krieger & Martin, 1981a). Also, some neurons have been identified as having receptors for multiple types of such neurotransmitters (Egan & North, 1981), and some neuropeptides apparently influence the release of other classes of neurotransmitters. For instance, Stefano, Hall, Markman, and Dvorkin (1981) found that neuropeptide opioids – which we will discuss in detail below – specifically and selectively inhibit the release of dopamine and norepinephrine, as well as other neurotransmitters, in regions of the mammalian central and peripheral nervous systems. Thus, the delineation of the role of both known and to-be-discovered neuropeptides is likely to provide major advances in knowledge of the function of the central nervous system. This potential benefit is highlighted by the recent observations that suggest that neurons have at least a constant, albeit low, level of expression of several peptides (Krieger & Martin, 1981a).

The endogenous opioids: endorphins and enkephalins

There are several major classes of neuropeptides: ACTH and the ACTH-like peptides, the neurohypophysical peptides (vasopressin and oxytocin), and the endogenous opioids – the endorphins and the enkephalins (Beatty, 1982). Although there are other types of neuropeptides (e.g., substance P), the endogenous opioids have been attracting most recent research attention (e.g., Bolles & Fanselow, 1982; Martinez, Jensen, Messing, Rigter, & McGaugh, 1981).

The identification of endogenous opiate-like substances in the brain is relatively recent (Bolles & Fanselow, 1982). Barchas and Sullivan (1982) summarize the history of the discovery of opioid peptide systems:

Among the most important contributions which led to the finding of endogenous opioids was the recognition that there might be opioid binding sites in the brain. Goldstein and his colleagues (1971) recognized this possibility, and their observations stimulated the search for such sites. Their ideas led to the discovery of opiate receptors by three independent groups, those of Terenius (1973), Simon (Simon et al., 1973), and Snyder (Pert & Snyder, 1973).
Another important direction that led to the recognition of endogenous opiates came from physiological studies dealing with stimulation-induced analgesia. These studies were highlighted in the investigations of Liebeskind and his group (1973, 1974). Akil performed studies demonstrating that naloxone, an opioid antagonist, reversed stimulation-induced analgesia (Akil et al., 1976). At that time, naloxone was believed to have no actions except the reversal of exogenous opiate effects. This observation then, along with the demonstration of receptors, suggested that there must be an endogenous opiate-like material. In what is already a classic set of studies, Hughes and Kosterlitz and their colleagues (Hughes et al., 1975) demonstrated the enkephalins. (Pp. 70–1)

Similarly, Bolles and Fanselow (1982, p. 88) recount that

there were indeed endogenous morphine-like agents, endorphins, residing there ("endorphin" is a contraction of endogenous and -orphine). The brain's opiates were part of a chain, the details of which had already been worked out. The segments Hughes had identified were positions 61 through 65 on the long polypeptide called β-lipotropin; they are usually designated met-enkephalin and leu-enkephalin. The other parts of β-lipotropin were well known. The first 41 positions of it is ACTH; the part in the middle, occupying positions 42 to 60, is the middle pituitary hormone MSH; the rest of it, 61 to 91 taken together, is designated β-endorphin, which had also been located in the pituitary.

However, although endogenous opiates have analgesic effects, as do opium derivatives such as morphine, the analgesic effect of beta-endorphin is 30 times greater than morphine, and another endorphin, dynorphin, is several hundred times more powerful (Thompson, 1981). Current research indicates that such action may occur, at least in part, because neuropeptides seem to generate rapid effects on neuronal membranes (Krieger & Martin, 1981a). Such neurotransmitters have relatively recently been synthesized, and so represent a potentially extremely useful means to treat pain in humans. This potential usefulness is bolstered by the findings of recent research suggesting that several methods used in the treatment of chronic pain – acupuncture, direct electrical stimulation of the brain, and hypnosis – act by promoting the release of endorphins and enkephalins (Iversen, 1979). This linkage is suggested by the finding that the effectiveness of all these chronic pain treatment methods can be blocked by the administration of naloxone, a chemical that blocks the binding of morphine to the opiate receptor and thus interferes with morphine's analgesic effects. Similarly, naloxone blocks the analgesic effects of beta-endorphin.

Research has also found that "opiate" receptors are present in those areas of the brain (especially, the ventrolateral periaqueductal gray matter of the midbrain) that produce analgesia in animals (Mayer, Wolfe, Akil, Carder, & Liebeskind, 1971) and humans (Hosobuchi, Adams, & Linchitz, 1977) when electrical stimulation is applied. Moreover, endorphins inhibit brain-stimulated distress vocalizations as well as pain (Herman & Panksepp, 1980). In addition, endogenous opiates are known to effect changes in mood and emotional behavior, although, whether it is an excess or a deficiency of endorphins that is involved in this effect is not certain (Marx, 1981d). Some studies find a lessening of psychotic symptoms upon administration of beta-endorphin, other studies find an increase in such symptoms, and there are a few studies that find no effect of administration (see Barchas & Sullivan, 1982 for a review). Despite the equivocal nature of this particular literature, most researchers still believe that there is a link between endogenous opiates and emotional disorders and that verification of the nature of this link will provide a crucial knowledge base for intervention (Barchas & Sullivan, 1982).

Other apparent roles for endorphins suggest several additional paths to intervention. Kunos, Farsang, and Ramirez-Gonzales (1981) report that beta-endorphin may facilitate the antihypertensive action of several drugs (e.g., clonidine and alpha-methyldopa). In turn, part of the pathophysiology of spinal cord injury is hypotension. Faden, Jacobs, and Holaday (1981) report that treatment with the opiate antagonist naloxone significantly improved the hypotension observed after cervical spinal trauma in cats, suggesting that endorphins are involved in the pathophysiology of spinal cord injury and that opiate antagonists may thus serve a therapeutic function in such cases.

Similarly, opiate antagonists may prove capable of playing a vital role in the treatment of stroke. Research by Hosobuchi, Baskin, and Woo (1982) illustrates this possibility. Homolateral cerebral ischemia and a neurologic deficit (stroke) were induced in 42% of a group of 140 adult male gerbils via microsurgical unilateral occlusion of the right common carotid artery. Intraperitoneal injection of naloxone reversed the signs of stroke within 3 to 5 minutes in all 10 of the affected gerbils tested. The effect of the naloxone lasted up to 30 minutes, after which stroke returned. However, repeated injections of naloxone were successful in continuing to reverse stroke. In addition, 9 other affected gerbils, implanted with small naloxone pellets, had continuous reversal of signs of stroke. Moreover, 24 gerbils that did not develop stroke after surgery were injected with morphine sulfate, and 21 developed stroke within 3 to 20 minutes. These strokes, which lasted from 4 to 24 hours, could be reversed by injection of naloxone.

The findings of Hosobuchi et al. (1982) suggest, as did the findings of Faden et al. (1981), the involvement of endorphins and opiate receptors in the pathophysiology of stroke. As in the case of spinal cord injury, the possibility arises of clinical use of opiate antagonists for treating injury to the organism – here for organisms in the acute phase of stroke (Hosobuchi et al., 1982). Regarding the potential use of endorphins for intervention in other types of physical trauma, Chernick and Craig (1982) found that endogenous opiates worsened neonatal depression caused by intrauterine asphyxia in rabbits, an effect that was reversed by naloxone.

In addition to the potential uses of endorphins for medical interventions, the endogenous opioids and several other neuropeptides have been, as noted above, linked to functions of perhaps greater concern to behavioral and social scientists. Since this latter connection not only provides a basis for a multilevel approach to research and intervention, but also illustrates the nature and bases of the plasticity of these neurotransmitters, we next focus on this connection.

Neuropeptides and behavioral and social functioning

The links between neuropeptides and behavior are complex and often contradictory ones (e.g., see Plomin & Deitrich, 1982), as recent scholarly reviews of data pertinent to the roles of such neurotransmitters in learning and memory have indicated (e.g., Martinez et al., 1981). However, there is evidence that opiate receptors are involved in specific aspects of rhesus monkey cortical function (Wise & Herbenhan, 1982) and that neuropeptides play a role in the memory of many species (e.g., rats), particularly when the memory involves aversively motivated instrumental responses. This latter success may be due to the presumed relation between the experience of fear and the release of neuropeptides such as endorphins (Bolles & Fanselow, 1982).

For example, Martinez and Rigter (1980) first gave rats passive avoidance training and then administered beta-endorphin, which resulted in a performance decrease on a subsequent test. Similarly, Iversen (1979) notes that administration of small amounts of the neuropeptide vasopressin have been found to result in significant improvements in laboratory animals' memory for aversively motivated learning tasks.

For example, hypophysectomized animals show impairment of conditioned avoidance behavior; however, this deficit is corrected by the administration of vasopressin as well as of some other peptide neurotransmitters – for example, alpha-MSH (Krieger & Martin, 1981b). Similar behavioral effects of these and other neuropeptides (e.g., alpha-endorphin) have been found in intact animals. Neuropeptides have been found to facilitate the rate of avoidance learning and, in turn, inhibit its extinction upon stimulus withdrawal (Krieger & Martin, 1981b).

As an indication of the rapid progress being made in the study of the role of these neurotransmitters in human functioning, consider that whereas Iversen in 1979 could only cite initial clinical work seeking to ascertain if vasopressin could facilitate remission in humans suffering from memory loss, by 1981 there was considerable evidence that it could. In a study by Weingartner et al. (1981) vasopressin was found to facilitate learning, as measured by the completeness, organization, and reliability of recall in both cognitively unimpaired and cognitively impaired adults. Vasopressin was also found useful in partially reversing the retrograde amnesia that follows electroconvulsive shock treatment. Similarly, vasopressin has been found to facilitate recovery of memory in patients with long-term amnesia resulting from car accidents (Oliveros et al., 1978) and to enhance attention and memory in the aged (Legros et al., 1978).

Neuropeptides other than vasopressin appear to be linked to cognitive functioning in the adult animal brain. Landfield, Baskin, and Pitler (1981) studied middle-aged rats who were either adrenalectomized and chronically maintained or were left intact and treated daily for a 9- to 10-month period with a potent analog of the peptide adrenocorticotropin or with the neural stimulant pentylenetetrazole. All three treatments reduced hippocampal morphologic correlates of brain aging (e.g., neuronal loss, glial reactivity). However, the pentylenetetrazole and the peptide treatments also improved learning response reversals. Landfield et al. conclude that certain endogenous peptides, with stimulant properties, may exert long-term trophic effects on brain structure and function. That is, as discussed in greater detail in Chapter 4 – for example, in the presentation of the work of Greenough (e.g., Greenough, 1975, 1978; Greenough & Green, 1981) – the adult brain is a plastic entity, the aging of the brain can be retarded, and the function of the brain (here in regard to a cognitive function) may be enhanced (here through a neurotransmitter-based intervention).

Another study of the role of opioids in aversively motivated learning not only underscores the links between neurotransmitters and behavioral functioning, but also leads to a broader discussion of the relation between the features of an organism's social context and its endogenous opiate production. Mauk, Warren, and Thompson (1982) found that intravenously administered morphine caused immediate and complete loss of a classically conditioned nictitating membrane extension response in rabbits and of the associated learning-induced increase in hippocampal neuron activity. The unconditioned stimulus used by Mauk et al. (1982) was an aversive one, a corneal airpuff. Given the role of opiates in abolishing memory of this aversively motivated simple learned response, the fact that the effects of morphine on this response and on neuron activity were completely reversed by naloxone, and the fact that morphine had no effect on the unconditioned response, led Mauk et al. to conclude that

some portion of the learned response – for memory retrieval of a simple, classically conditioned response to an aversive [unconditioned stimulus] – is impaired by morphine. It may be that conditioned aversiveness or fear is an essential component of learning and memory in this task. Considerable evidence implicates morphine as acting on conditioned fear. (Pp. 435–6)

Other evidence linking environmentally induced aversive-learning or fearlike states to the production of endogenous opiates derives from the research of Miczek, Thompson, and Shuster (1982), a study that also illustrates the link between social context variables and intraindividual endogenous opiate production. Miczek et al. exposed mice to repeated attacks by other mice. This exposure led to a decrease in nociception in response to radiant heat focused on the tails of the attacked mice. This form of analgesia was blocked, however, by naloxone. In addition, among those mice who were repeatedly subjected to defeat, analgesia after morphine administration was much less than was the case among those mice not subjected to defeat. Underscoring the complex, socially embedded nature of this endogenous opiate production in the defeated mice, Miczek et al. (p. 1522) point out that

defeat in a social confrontation is stressful and engenders analgesia. Yet, attacking mice show no increase in tail-flick latencies, even though they receive occasional retaliatory bites by the intruders and experience substantial pituitary-adrenal activation while attacking. Apparently, the special biological significance of the defeat experience, and not simply the experience of being stressed, is critical to the occurrence of opioid-like analgesia.

Additional support for a link between endogenous opiates and social contextual functions derives from research by Panksepp et al. (1978) and by Herman and Panksepp (1980) suggesting that alteration of social relationships leads to alteration of opioid peptide levels. Both studies report that loss of social relationships – interpreted as a state of social distress – resulted in an increase in endogenous opiate levels, which in turn led to a decrement in social distress (Herman & Panksepp, 1980; Panksepp et al., 1978). These data thus provide evidence that contextual variables alter brain neurochemistry and that, in turn, the neurochemicals change the organism's psychological functioning.

Similar connections can be inferred from data reported by Madden, Akil, Patrick, and Barchas (1977). After rats were stressed, increased concentrations of opioid peptides were found in their brains; concomitant with this change was a congruent change in the organism's functioning, specifically, an increase in pain threshold.

Highlighting the link between social behavior and endogenous opiate production, and thus the potential appropriateness of collaborative research by behavioral and neuroscientists, are data suggesting that the normal onset and maintenance of maternal behavior may be moderated by endogenous opiates. Bridges and Grimm (1982) surgically terminated the pregnancies of rats on day 17 of gestation. The rats were then injected with morphine, with morphine plus naloxone, or with saline. All rats were then tested for maternal responsiveness toward foster-young. There was a significant disruption of the rate of onset and of the quality of maternal responsiveness among the rats treated with morphine alone. However, among the rats treated with both naloxone and morphine, there was a rapid onset of behavioral responsiveness toward the foster-young. In fact, the behavior of this naloxone-plus-morphine group toward the foster-young was indistinguishable from that seen among the saline-injected control rats.

Finally, another line of evidence may be noted to illustrate the links between endogenous opiate production and contextual variables. This line of research additionally illustrates the plasticity of endogenous opiate production processes – here in terms of how contextual variables may become linked with, and indeed enter into, the control of such processes. Lastly, this line of research suggests that the organism itself may contribute, in a self-regulatory sense, to these processes.

Watkins and Mayer (1982) have reviewed evidence that demonstrates that endorphin-mediated, pain-modulating mechanisms in the CNS can be environmentally activated (e.g., through foot shock). Moreover, they report that the study of such "foot-shock-induced analgesia" (FSIA) reflects plasticity in analgesic systems and that such plasticity involves the organism's molar, behavioral self-regulation. Hayes, Bennett, Newlon, and Mayer (1978) found that by use of a classical conditioning paradigm, rats could be shown to associate environmental cues with shock delivery. More important here, however, the rats

learned to activate their endogenous pain-inhibitory systems when these cues were presented. In that study, the nonelectrified shock chamber was the conditioned stimulus (CS), grid shock delivered to all four paws was the unconditioned stimulus (UCS), and tail-flick inhibition was the unconditioned response (UCR). After CS–UCS pairings, exposure to the nonelectrified grid reliably induced analgesia. (Watkins & Mayer, 1982, p. 1188)

Furthermore, since Watkins and Mayer (1982) demonstrated that rat front paw FSIA is mediated through a well-defined opiate pathway in the brain, they used brief front paw shock as the UCS in a classical conditioning study in order to determine whether plasticity exists in opiate systems; that is, they assessed whether the rats could learn to activate their endogenous opiate systems to inhibit pain; in other words, they determined if the control of the endogenous opiate system could be altered from organism-independent environmental stimulus to organism-dependent learning. Their results indicated this to be the case:

Exposure to the nonelectrified grid (CS) produced potent analgesia after being paired with front paw shock. The observation that classically conditioned analgesia can be antagonized by systemic naloxone,... spinal naloxone, and morphine tolerance suggests that animals learn to activate an endogenous opiate system. Maintenance of the analgesic state again seems to be independent of continued opiate release. As with front paw FSIA, we have observed that naloxone can prevent, but cannot reverse, classically conditioned analgesia.

Although opiate (front paw) and non-opiate (hind paw) FSIA can be differentially elicited, classically conditioned analgesia seems always to involve opiate pathways regardless of the body region shocked during conditioning trials. Classically conditioned analgesia can be antagonized by naloxone regardless of whether front paw or hind paw shock is used as the UCS. (Watkins & Mayer, 1982, pp. 1188–9)

Thus, the Watkins and Mayer (1982) data, as well as those of Miczek et al. (1982), suggest a link between the active organism and neuropeptide production; that is, the learning and interacting organism is part of the process producing its own neuropeptides. This link between the organism's behavioral and neurochemical levels not only highlights the need for a multilevel approach to research and intervention. In addition, it suggests that the relations among levels may best be viewed as a bidirectional one, one involving plastic processes. These views are supported by additional data pertinent to the role of the organism (e.g., its cognition, perception, and behavioral repertoire) as part of the process by which neuropeptides may be produced. That is, not only do brain chemicals affect cognition and behavior but, in turn, cognitive and behavioral functioning apparently impact on chemical production.

Levine, Gordon, and Fields (1978) present data indicating that placebo administration with humans is sufficient to elevate endorphin levels in the blood. Levine et al. (1978) studied patients undergoing treatment for dental postoperative pain. Endogenous opiates may be expected to produce analgesia response to such pain. Indeed, the fact that the patients to whom Levine et al. administered naloxone reported an increase in pain supports such a view of the role of endorphins. However, the ability of cognition to control endorphin release is suggested by the fact that among those patients for whom administration of a placebo decreased pain, subsequent administration of naloxone increased pain, although among patients for whom placebo administration did not decrease pain, subsequent naloxone administration did not increase pain. These data suggest that endorphin release mediates placebo analgesia (Levine et al., 1978), that is, if one believes a chemically neutral drug will reduce pain, this cognition is sufficient to release endorphins sufficient to diminish pain, at least insofar as postoperative dental pain is concerned.

Data reported by Willer, Dehen, and Cambier (1981) provide additional support for the role of humans' cognitive functioning in neuropeptide production, here in regard to learning an aversively motivated task and to perception; in addition, the Willer et al. (1981) data lead us to a discussion of the role of contextual events that stress the organism in neuropeptide production. Willer et al. note that the psychological conditions of stress and anxiety can modify the perception of pain and spinal excitability. They report that endogenous opioids are involved in the phenomenon of stress-induced analgesia in normal men and women. To demonstrate this they assessed the cumulative effects of a repetitive stress, induced by anticipation of pain (noxious foot shock), on the threshold of a nociceptive flexion reflex of the lower limb. The threshold of the reflex progressively increased with the repetition of the stress; endogenous opioids were implicated in this change since the threshold-elevating effect of the stress was reversed by naloxone, which even produced hyperalgesia (i.e., a rapid and significant decrease in the threshold below the initial values was noted).

From data such as that reported by Willer et al. (1981) it appears that humans can tolerate and adapt to repeated, perhaps even increased, levels of stress as a consequence of endogenous opioid production. While such a process may be quite useful when the person is faced with a situation calling for intense confrontation with a stressor (e.g., in battle, in games involving prolonged physical exertion), not all instances of the functioning of such a process may be beneficial. If we recall that the addictive effects of endogenous opiates may be considerably more powerful than exogenous ones, then it is possible that people, once placed in particular stress producing situations, come to place themselves in such settings in order to produce endogenous opiates.

Evidence for the presence of such a process may be found in animal research. In a study of exposure of rats to a series of inescapable shocks, Grau et al. (1981) found that the activation of opiate systems is necessary and sufficient to produce long-term stress-induced analgesia (SIA) and that opiates and inescapable shock share some common action in that both activate the effectiveness of endogenous opiates.

Instances of this mechanism in humans may be involved in what is often labeled "thrill-seeking" behaviors, and Thompson (1981) suggests that it may also be involved in compulsive gambling; he notes that a possible intervention in such stress-induced behavior is the administration of naloxone. Data reported by Morley and Levine (1981) that support Thompson's view relate to stress in rats induced by tail pinching. Such stress induction is associated with eating, which in turn apparently involves the endogenous opiods because Morley and Levine (1981) found that naloxone attenuated such stress-induced eating. In addition to such remedial, pharmacological intervention one could use behavior and cognitive–behavior therapies (Kendall, 1981) as preventive and/or remedial intervention. Humans can conceivably acquire skills to avoid or alter situations that produce stress and thus induce endogenous opioid production; cognitive strategies (e.g., verbal self-instructions, cognitive restructuring, labeling) could be useful in allowing the person to redefine the situation and/or alter his or her behavior. By thus avoiding or at least altering escalation of the "stress→endogenous opioid production→changed threshold" sequence, behavioral and cognitive–behavioral interventions may be useful in treating what can be labeled "addictive stress situations," as, for example, those involved in compulsive gambling or compulsive eating. Such psychological interventions would enable individuals to control the effects of stressors without recourse to pharmacological treatments; acquisition of such "stress management" abilities would allow people to function more effectively in situations where unanticipated stressors are the norm.

Conclusions

The interrelations between brain chemicals and behaviors provide several indications that fertile and important multidisciplinary research and intervention can be conducted. Further research and intervention among neurochemists and developmental and cognitive psychologists may seek to answer questions such as "Which neurotransmitters, among what populations, studied at what age levels, may moderate or enhance which cognitive functions (as indexed by what measures)?" As we proceed, in the following chapters, to examine variables and processes at levels more molar than is neurochemistry, we will see that plasticity continues to be a key feature of organism functioning and that multidisciplinary research and intervention efforts promise to be useful at these levels as well.

6 Evolutionary biology and hominid evolution

Several lines of evidence, derived from the literatures of evolutionary biology and anthropology, converge in suggesting that (1) features of human macro-evolutionary change and of human microevolution provided a structural contribution to the unique degree of plasticity that characterizes humans' processes of development; (2) this evolution was both a basis of and derived from humans' behavioral, social, and cultural development; and (3) as a consequence, biological functioning and change – in regard to both ontogenetic and evolutionary progressions – are reciprocally related, first, to the social and cultural forces acting on the organism and, second, to the organism's own behavior as well. In this view, then, not only, for instance, did the evolution of the human brain enable humans to be socially responsive, but at the same time humans' social and cultural embeddedness were the key selection features for the human brain. In other words, human plasticity derives from an evolutionary synthesis between the human brain and human culture (Gould, 1977; Masters, 1978; Washburn, 1961).

Although work in support of these links has a long history, indeed dating back to at least the early nineteenth century, two lines of evidence will be presented. The first line of evidence derives from a recent, comprehensive scholarly integration of the literatures relevant to the concept of heterochrony (or differences in timing) in human evolution and development. This synthesis has been presented by Gould in his highly influential book *Ontogeny and Phylogeny* (1977). I rely greatly on Gould's work in presenting my own, not only because of the thoroughness and soundness of Gould's presentation but also because his ideas have critical relevance for the integrations I am attempting to make in this book. Specifically, I will argue that Gould's (1977) integration has importance for two other areas of scholarship bearing on the study of human plasticity and on its significance for multidisciplinary research and intervention: the comparative–developmental psychological and the sociological – intergenerational areas of scholarship. I will indicate in this chapter how Gould's (1977) contribution converges with evidence from comparative physical anthropological and paleoanthropological research, and reserve for succeeding chapters a discussion of how Gould's ideas about heterochrony relate to comparative–developmental psychological and sociological intergenerational research pertinent to plasticity.

The second line of evidence pertinent to evolutionary biology and human evolution that I will review in this chapter is also associated with the work of Gould. Here, however, we will consider how the problems posed by attempting to understand the relations between marcroevolutionary and microevolutionary processes may be addressed by revising the concepts used to speak about adaptation and fitness. Gould and Vrba (1982) suggest we revise the terms used to discuss organism fitness, and in so doing not only help integrate microevolutionary (genomic evolutionary) processes and macroevolutionary processes (those that pertain to the origins of species diversity), but in addition show how the processes involved in this integration may provide a basis of human evolutionary plasticity.

Let us begin our discussion by turning first to the contributions Gould has made to clarifying the relations betwen ontogeny and phylogeny.

Heterochrony in evolution and development

As evident from the title of his book, Gould's (1977) interest is in detailing the relation between ontogeny and phylogeny. He states: "That some relationship exists cannot be denied. Evolutionary changes must be expressed in ontogeny, and phyletic information must therefore reside in the development of individuals" (p. 2). However this point, in itself, is obvious and unenlightening for Gould. What makes the study of the relation between ontogeny and phylogeny interesting and important is that there are "*changes* in *developmental timing* that produce *parallels* between the stages of ontogeny and phylogeny" (p. 2).

However, to discuss the relation between ontogeny and phylogeny may "raise the hackles" (read: Haeckel's) of many scientists. This may be especially true for those trained in developmental psychology, where the recapitulationist ideas of Haeckel (e.g., 1868), especially as they were adopted by G. S. Hall (1904), have long been in disfavor. In simplified form, Haeckel's theory was one of *recapitulation*, by which he meant that the mechanism of evolution was *a change in the timing of developmental events such that there occurred a universal acceleration of development that pushed ancestral forms into the juvenile stages of descendants* (Gould, 1977). For example, Haeckel (1868) interpreted the gill slits of human embryos as characteristics of ancestral adult fishes that had been compressed into the early stages of human ontogeny through a universal mechanism of acceleration of developmental rates in evolving lines.

It is unfortunate for the scientific study of links between ontogeny and phylogeny that people have come to equate Haeckel's concept of recapitulation with all potential types and directions of evolutionary change in the timing of developmental events. This is because there is an alternative to the changes in timing specified by recapitulation. To Gould, this alternative is the key to human evolution and to human plasticity. To understand this alternative we need to introduce three interrelated terms: heterochrony, neoteny, and paedomorphosis.

According to Gould, evolution occurs when ontogeny is altered in one of two ways: (1) when new characteristics are introduced at any stage of development, which then have varying influences on later developmental stages; and (2) when characteristics that are already present undergo changes in developmental timing. This second means by which phyletic change occurs is termed *heterochrony*. Specifically, heterochrony describes the situation wherein changes occur in the relative time of appearance and rate of development of characteristics already present in ancestors (Gould, 1977, p. 2).

Human evolution has resulted in a specific type of heterochrony for the species, one that has resulted in the changes associated with human plasticity. The type of heterochrony that has characterized human evolution is *neoteny*, which is a slowing down, a retardation of development for selected somatic organs and parts (Gould, 1977, p. 9). Heterochronic changes are regulatory effects, that is, they constitute "a change in rate for features already present" (p. 8). Gould maintains that neoteny has been a major determinant, and probably *the* major determinant, of human evolution.

For example, as explained in greater detail below, delayed growth has been found to be important in the evolution of complex and flexible social behavior, and, interrelatedly, it has led to an increase in cerebralization by prolonging into later human life the rapid brain growth characteristics of other higher vertebrate fetuses (Gould, 1977, p. 9). This general evolutionary retardation of human development has resulted in the retention of adaptive features of ancestral juveniles. That is, a key characteristic of human evolution is *paedomorphosis*, or phylogenetic change involving retention of ancestral juvenile charcteristics by the adult. In other words:

Our paedomorphic features are a set of adaptations coordinated by their common efficient cause of retarded development. We are not neotenous only because we possess an impressive set of paedomorphic characters; we are neotenous because these characters develop within a matrix of retarded development that coordinates their common appearance in human adults.... [These] temporal delays themselves are the most significant feature of human heterochrony. (Pp. 397, 399)

What are these paedomorphic–neotenous characteristics? How do they provide an evolutionary basis of human plasticity? Gould himself answers these questions, and in so doing indicates that humans' evolving plasticity both enabled and resulted from their embeddedness in a social and cultural context. He states:

In asserting the importance of delayed development ... I assume that major human adaptations acted synergistically throughout their gradual development.... *The inter-acting system of delayed development–upright posture–large brain is such a complex:* delayed development has produced a large brain by prolonging fetal growth rates and has supplied a set of cranial proportions adapted to upright posture. Upright posture freed the hand for tool use and set selection pressures for an expanded brain. A large brain may, itself entail a longer life span.... Human evolution has *emphasized* one feature of ... common primate heritage – delayed development, particularly as expressed in late instruction and extended childhood. This retardation has reacted synergistically with other hallmarks of hominization – with intelligence (by enlarging the brain through prolongation of fetal growth tendencies and by providing a longer period of childhood learning) and with socialization (by cementing family units through increased parental care of slowly developing offspring). *It is hard to imagine how the distinctive suite of human characters could have emerged outside the context of delayed development.* (Pp. 399, 400; italics added)

Thus, in linking neoteny with reciprocal relations between brain development and sociocultural functioning, Gould makes an argument of extreme importance for comparative–developmental and sociocultural–intergenerational analyses of human development. The role of the former type of analysis is addressed in regard to species differences (heterochrony) in the ontogeny of brain organization and to their import for levels of plasticity finally attained across life; the role of the latter type of analysis is addressed in regard to the role of parent–child relations in promoting the child's development toward a final level of functioning characterized by plasticity. As noted earlier, we will consider these implications for comparative–developmental and sociocultural–intergenerational analyses of human development and plasticity, respectively, in the next two chapters. Here, however, it is important to note that in other portions of the evolutionary biology literature, and in the anthropology literature, there is support for the link suggested by Gould between plastic brain development and human sociocultural functioning.

Longevity and neoteny: comparative physical anthropological evidence

A perspective on human neoteny compatible with Gould's (1977) is provided by Washburn (1981), whose analysis draws on comparative data on both extant primate species and the hominid fossil record. Washburn's perspective will lead us to a consideration of paleoanthropological information pertinent to Gould's ideas about the role of neoteny in human evolution.

In discussing longevity in primates, Washburn notes that one may divide the life span into three phases in order to make comparisons among species. The first phase, termed *preparation*, pertains to the length of time it takes for the species to mature. The second phase, *adaptation*, denotes the length of time adults are biologically adapted to the problems of living effectively. The third

Table 1. *Length of phases of primate life-span in years*

Primate species	Preparation			Adaptation	Decline
	Eruption of first molars	Eruption of second molars	Eruption of third molars		
Macaque	2	4	6	6–20	20–35
Chimpanzee	3	6	10	10–30	30–50
Human	6	12	18	18–45	45–75

Source: Adapted from Washburn (1981, p. 13).

phase, *decline*, denotes the longevity of some individual members of the species under optimal environmental conditions.

Washburn stresses two points about these life-span phases. First, each phase is differentially related to species survival. He notes that:

for selection to favor long infant and juvenile periods, those periods must result in the greater reproductive success of adults. Reproductive success in the second period determines the evolutionary success of the species, and the third period is a by-product.

That is (in regard to the third phase):

Viewing old age as a by-product of adaptation at younger ages helps to explain why the rates of aging may be so different in different individuals. As Lapin, Krilova, Cherkovich, and Asanov (1979, p. 35) have stated, "There is often no correlation between the manifestations of aging in different systems." Evolution shows why this is the case. High correlations are the result of selection, and there never was selection for healthy old people. The old were already dead before their genes could affect the course of human evolution. (P. 27)

The second point Washburn makes about these three life-span phases is that "in contemporary human beings, each phase is much longer than in any other primate" (p. 13). Table 1, adapted from Washburn (1981), illustrates this point. The length of years spent in each of the three life-span phases is shown for each of three primate species: the macaque, the chimpanzee, and the human. The preparation phase in each species is compared on the basis of the age at which the first, second, and third molars appear. All three phases are longer for humans than for the other two primate species.

Washburn argues that the differences between the brains of apes and human beings cannot be understood if the only features assessed are variables such as brain size or weight. He notes that human technical skills, social effectiveness, and linguistic abilities, which are made possible by the human brain, are comparatively new in evolution, and he believes that humans' neotenous evolutionary rates – which correlate with these new functions – are also evolutionarily new;

they are not merely the continuations of rates persisting from the long-distant past.

Direct evidence for this comes from the analysis of the development of teeth. As indicated in Table 1, Washburn notes that the eruption of the permanent teeth has slowed in humans. For instance, the second molar does not show in an X-ray at the time the first molar erupts, and a similar relation exists in regard to the second and third molars. A similar maturational sequence existed in australopithecines. In contrast, however, in apes when a tooth has erupted the tooth that will erupt next is already calcified (Washburn, 1981). The neotenous character of human development is thus illustrated by the delay in human tooth eruption time, a delay identified by recourse to data derived from a comparative analysis of tooth maturation. Moreover, this analysis – including data pertinent to comparisons of humans with both other extant primate species and with extinct species in the fossil record – leads us to a more general consideration of paleoanthropological evidence pertinent to Gould's (1977) views.

Bidirectional organism–context relations in evolution:
paleoanthropological perspectives

Current anthropological theory suggests that humans have been selected for social dependency: The course and context of evolution was such that it was more adaptive to act in concert, with the group, than in isolation. For example, Masters (1978) notes that early hominids were hunters. These ancestors evolved from herbivorous primates under the pressure of climatic changes that caused the African forest to be replaced with savannah. Our large brains, he speculates (p. 98), may be the (naturally selected) result of cooperation among early hominids and hence, in an evolutionary sense, a social organ. Indeed, he believes that identifying this aspect of human evolution may help solve the "central problem" in anthropological analysis, that of the origin of human society. Washburn (1961) appears to agree. He notes that the relative defenselessness of early humans (lack of fighting teeth, nails, or horns), coupled with the dangers of living on the open African savannah, made group living and cooperation essential for survival (Washburn, 1961; see also Hogan, Johnson, & Emler, 1978).

There is some dispute in modern anthropological theory as to whether material culture or specific features of social relations, such as intensified parenting, monogamous pair bonding, nuclear family formation, and thus specialized sexual-reproductive behavior, were superordinate in these brain–behavior evolutionary relations. For example, paleoanthropologists currently believe that there are five characteristics that separate humans from other hominids: a large neocortex, bipedality, reduced anterior dentation with molar dominance, material culture, and unique sexual and reproductive behavior (e.g., of all primates only the human female's sexual behavior is not confined to the middle of her monthly menstrual cycle; Fisher, 1982a). Some paleoanthropologists believe that early human evolution was a direct consequence of brain expansion and material culture. However, Lovejoy (1981), among others (e.g., Johanson & Edey, 1981) believes that

both advanced material culture and the Pleistocene acceleration in brain development are sequelae to an already established hominid character system, which included intensified parenting and social relationships, monogamous pair bonding, specialized sexual–reproductive behavior, and bipedality. (P. 348)

Other theoretical debates concern, for instance, the complex roles played by continual sexual receptivity and loss of estrus in the evolution of human pair bonding (e.g., Fisher, 1982b; Harley, 1982; Isaac, 1982; Swartz, 1982; Washburn, 1982).

Such debate, however, exists in the midst of the general consensus indicated above – that the social functioning of hominids (be it interpreted as dyadic, familial, or cultural) was reciprocally related to the evolution of the human brain. Many evolutionary biologists appear to reach a similar conclusion.

For example, summarizing the literature pertaining to the character of the environment to which organisms adapt, Lewontin and Levins (1978) stress that reciprocal processes between organism and environment are involved in human evolution, supporting the view that human functioning is one source of its own evolutionary development. Lewontin and Levins (1978, p. 78) state that

the activity of the organism sets the stage for its own evolution. . . . the labor process by which the human ancestors modified natural objects to make them suitable for human use was itself the unique feature of the way of life that directed selection on the hand, larynx, and brain in a positive feedback that transformed the species, its environment, and its mode of interaction with nature.

Lovejoy (1981) and Fisher (1982a), both graphically recounting the history of the role of hominid social behavior in human evolution, lend support to Gould's (1977) views by showing how the complex social and physical facets of this evolution led to human neoteny. Interestingly, while Fisher and (especially) Lovejoy tend to view the ecological influences that led to the evolution of social behaviors as eventuating in bipedalism and then rapid brain development, they nevertheless both see these links in more of a circular than a linear framework.

To illustrate, Fisher (1982a) notes that 14 million years ago, hominids were already exploring the expanding African woodlands and grasslands. During this period, hominids stopped living exclusively in trees and began to travel quadrupedally into the woodlands in order to forage among the low-limbed trees. Extrapolating from the fact that chimpanzees use tools regularly, Fisher speculates that the most intelligent of these hominids may have used sticks and stones as such implements in order to pry up roots or smash nuts. In any event, she believes it is likely that at this time hominids began to coordinate efforts to hunt small animals, since such behavior would increase the likelihood of each member of the group gaining access to food and since such "tolerated scrounging" is common among chimpanzees and baboons. Thus, the dependence of the individual on the group was supported by the enhanced likelihood that such social embeddedness would lead to more food.

Moreover, because the woodlands were then dangerous for relatively defenseless hominids (e.g., there was an abundance of leopards and other large cats sharing the setting), and because the ecology itself was significantly changing (fewer trees, with lower limbs, spaced farther apart), two adaptational solutions arose (Fisher, 1982a). Again reinforcing the social embeddedness of the individual, hominids began to travel in small, cohesive groups in order to protect themselves. Second, sticks and stones were picked up and thrown as "defensive tools"; thus, a second basis for tool use emerged. Despite this growing group cohesion, Fisher believes there was no heterosexual pair bonding. Instead, females had a monthly period of heat and males competed for the attention of estrous females. Moreover, it is not likely, Fisher believes, that at this time males aided females in caring for the young.

When, by about 8 million years ago, the woodlands were evolving into savannas, a major change was fostered among our hominid ancestors, one that led quite directly to the human neotenous brain. Fisher describes this crucial change as follows:

Gradually, during the dry seasons, small groups of protohominids – the branch of hominids that leads to humans – must have been forced onto the plains, where life was even more dangerous; there were more open spaces, and even fewer trees to climb. By day, protohominids must have banded together, sleeping in trees or in protected, dried-up streambeds at night. At this juncture, a major innovation occurred: Because of the dangers of savanna living, it seems likely that individuals soon discovered the practicality of gathering vegetables or small mammals and quickly carrying them back to a central location – perhaps to where they had slept the night before. They probably also discovered that sticks and stones were no longer available every time they needed them, and that it was more practical to tote them as well. The innovation, of course, was carrying, and in order to carry efficiently they had to walk bipedally.

Because bipedalism was essential to survival in the savanna, it seems likely that this new upright stance evolved rapidly. Protohominids would never have evolved other human characteristics – such as bonding, kinship, language, culture, or a highly developed brain – if not for bipedalism. It is well known that bipedalism led, of necessity, to major changes in the hominid skeleton. It seems a forgotten point, however, that a byproduct of that anatomical revolution was a reduction in the size of one, and perhaps two, major diameters of the pelvic inlet – the birth canal. (Fisher, 1982a, p. 20)

This change in the birth canal provided a key basis for human neoteny. The effect of reducing the birth canal's diameter would create obstetrical difficulties, for the head of the hominid fetus would be too large to pass through it. In 1960 Washburn indicated that this obstetrical difficulty could have been solved by the fetus being delivered at an earlier stage of development (Fisher, 1982a). Fisher believes it is likely that

among protohominids, there were a few females with the genetic ability to bear their young at an earlier stage. Normally this would have been a deleterious trait. However, at this critical moment in protohominid history, those females who bore premature infants (whose heads could easily navigate the shrinking birth canal) would have survived and so would have their young. Thus these females disproportionately bred, and slowly the genetic trait for premature parturition predominated among females of the protohominid population. (P. 20)

Thus, in hominids born prematurely, development that would have occurred in the less stimulative in utero environment occurred outside the womb. A selection for slower (neotenous) in utero brain growth led to a trajectory of hominid evolution wherein ontogenetic changes previously completed before birth were extended well into the years following birth. That is, as Gould (1977) has indicated, humans have evolved to be born with ''immature'' brains, brains that undergo continued development perhaps across the life span. Moreover, ''solutions'' involving neoteny simultaneously further promoted social embeddedness and especially pair bonding. To return once again to the account of Fisher (1982a, p. 20), the presence of premature young left females with infants

requiring many extra weeks, even months, of care. Morever, because mothers now walked bipedally, they had to carry their infants in their arms instead of on their backs. Females must have found it increasingly difficult to ... chase after small animals and [join] hunting parties. Gone were the days when protohominid females could independently cope with their young.

To survive the female needed a mate, at least for the period, following birth of the infant, when the mother was least able to fend for herself. Because of this need, Fisher believes, consort relationships were developed. And such relationships were not only advantageous to the mother and infant, but to the male as well:

Certainly an extended consortship provided tremendous benefits to females, but consorts may have been appealing to protohominid males as well – particularly in the dry season. By traveling with a mate, a male could share the nuts of one bush, the fruit of one tree, the eggs of one nest, and move on without waiting for a larger group. If he found no meat, he could depend on her to gather vegetables. During the consortship, he would not have had to compete with other males for sexual access to the female. Moreover, although he was unaware of it, if he attended to the offspring he sired by this female, they might live to pass on his genes. Thus males with even a slight predisposition to bond – to form an extended consortship – bred more, produced more offspring, and more of their young survived – spreading to each succeeding generation a disproportionate number of genes of both males and females with a tendency to bond.
 In this fashion, bonding spread through the protohominid population. (Fisher, 1982a, p. 21)

Thus, Fisher (1982a) describes a complex set of evolutionary relationships among variables pertinent to physical ecology, social relationship development, physical and physiological changes, and pair bonding – all of which coalesced to create a neotenous human, one embedded in a social context in a reciprocal manner. Although the evolutionary relationships Fisher describes are in the main consistent with Lovejoy's (1981) ideas about the importance of social relationships, she presents them as if they evolved in a linear manner, whereas Lovejoy (1981), in agreement with Lewontin and Levins (1978), sees these relationships in a reciprocal framework. That is, it is not just that ecological changes led to social relationships, which in turn led to bipedalism and, in turn, to brain evolution. Instead, social relationships that led to brain evolution were then themselves altered when larger-brained – and more plastic – organisms were involved in them; in turn, new social patterns may have extended humans' functioning into other arenas, ones fostering further changes in the brain, in social embeddedness, and so forth. Thus, Johanson and Edey (1981) describe Lovejoy's position as one requiring the examination of

the mechanism of a complex feedback loop – in which several elements interact for mutual reinforcement. . . . If parental care is a good thing, it will be selected for by the likelihood that the better mothers will be more apt to bring up children, and thus intensify any genetic tendency that exists in the population toward being better mothers. But increased parental care requires other things along with it. It requires a greater IQ on the part of the mother; she cannot increase parental care if she is not intellectually up to it. That means brain development – not only for the mother, but for the infant daughter too, for someday she will become a mother.

In the case of primate evolution, the feedback is not just a simple A-B stimulus forward and backward between two poles. It is multi-poled and circular, with many features to it instead of only two – all of them mutually reinforcing. For example, if an infant is to have a large brain, it must be given time to learn to use that brain before it has to face the world on its own. That means a long childhood. The best way to learn during childhood is to play. That means playmates, which, in turn, means a group social system that provides them. But if one is to function in such a group, one must learn acceptable social behavior. One can learn that properly only if one is intelligent. Therefore social behavior ends up being linked with IQ (a loop back), with extended childhood (another loop), and finally with the energy investment and the parental care system which provide a brain capable of that IQ, and the entire feedback loop is complete.

All parts of the feedback system are cross-connected. For example: if one is living in a group, the time spent finding food, being aware of predators and finding a mate can all be reduced by the very fact that one is in a group. As a consequence, more time can be spent on parental care (one loop), on play (another) and on social activity (another), all of which enhance intelligence (another) and result ultimately in fewer offspring (still another). The complete loop shows all poles connected to all others. (Pp. 325–6)

This "complete loop," or system of reciprocal influence, is illustrated in Figure 1, showing the foundations of human plasticity evolved in a complex system of bidirectional relationships among social, ontogenetic, and neuronal variables.

A comparable system of bidirectional relations emerges from the research and writing of Robert Martin. Martin also indicates that the human postnatal growth

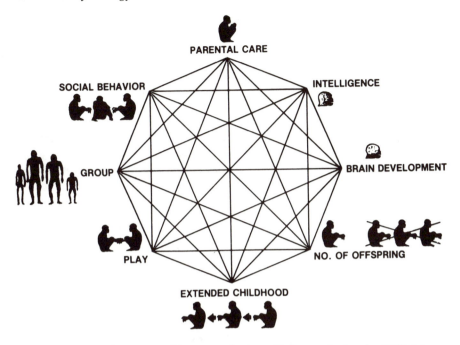

Figure 1. Components of the system of reciprocal influences that Lovejoy (1981; Johanson & Edey, 1981) believes was involved in the evolution of human neoteny and social embeddedness (Adapted from Johanson & Edey, 1981, p. 327.)

period is something unique among primates (in Lewin, 1982b) and places evolution of the large human brain in a system of relations that includes human reproductive strategy, the elaboration of culture (e.g., in regard to eating and feeding behaviors), and the features of the physical ecology within which hominid evolution occurred. Martin (in Lewin, 1982b) contrasts two general types of reproductive strategy: r-selection and K-selection. With r-selection mammals generally produce large litters whereas with a K-selection reproductive strategy typically one, and rarely more than three, offspring are produced per birth experience.

Martin (quoted in Lewin, 1982b, p. 840) notes that

r-selection is suited to unstable environments where for a lot of the time populations will be in a growth phase. You have selection for high reproductive output and little for efficiency of resource utilization in these circumstances. By contrast, K-selection is effective in stable environments in which populations are mostly close to carrying capacity. In this case, there is selection for high efficiency in use of resources and low reproductive output.

The implication of Martin's view is that hominids evolved in a stable (i.e., K-selection) environment and adopted ''a high energy feeding strategy that would have sustained the development of a large brain'' (quoted in Lewin, 1982b, p. 841). That this occurred, Martin believes, is evidenced by the fact that human infants have brains and bodies twice as big as one would expect given the length of gestation and because "this must be extremely costly energetically . . . a high energy feeding strategy was essential for . . . development'' (Martin, 1982, quoted in Lewin, 1982b, p. 841).

While rain forests would have provided the stable environment necessary for this K-selection and associated evolution, there is a general consensus (as evidenced, e.g., in Fisher's [1982a] work) that early hominid evolution shifted relatively early to the savanna. Martin does not dispute this view, but believes that this shift involves the contribution of human culture. That is, if humans

were living on the savanna they would have had to adopt cultural techniques with which to even out the erratic supply of food. The use of digging sticks to gain access to energy-rich tubers would be a good example. (Quoted in Lewin, 1982b, p. 841)

Conclusions

Our analysis of Gould's ideas pertinent to the role of neotenous heterochrony in the evolution of human plasticity has led us to a discussion of the role of reciprocal relations between organisms and their contexts in human evolution. It is important to point out that the explanation of the evolution of human plasticity that has emerged from this presentation is one that stresses the systemic, probabilistic-epigenetic nature of change. In other words, the properties that have evolved to characterize the human system – that is, humans' relations with their context – are not those that might be inferred by studying the parts of the system in isolation. The evolutionary biologist Ernst Mayr, for instance, takes a stance consistent with the contextual, probabilistic causal framework that, we noted in Chapters 1 and 2, is today emerging in biological and social science (e.g., Gottlieb, 1970; Schneirla, 1957; Sperry, 1982a) and to which we have been led to in this chapter. Mayr states:

New properties turn up in systems that could not have been predicted from the components, which means you have to study things hierarchically. Reductionism can be vacuous at best, and, in the face of emergence, misleading and futile. . . . We simply claim that in complex, historically formed systems things occur that do not occur in inanimate systems. (Quoted in Lewin, 1982a, p. 720).

Maynard-Smith (1982) makes a quite similar point, noting that

although at the molecular level a single process often turns out to have a single cause, unitary explanations are less commonly true at the organismic level. There are general principles in evolutionary biology, notably the principle of natural selection, but the details of the process are irreducibly complex. (Maynard-Smith, 1982, p. 382)

Thus, Mayr (1982) believes that biology expands the limits of the philosophy of science beyond those defined by the physical sciences. That is, "not only are biological systems too complex to admit of simple reductionism; they are too diverse to admit of universal laws and can be described only by 'probabilistic' generalizations to which there invariably will be exceptions" (Futuyma, 1982, p. 833).

In sum, biological adaptation means social adaptation; in other words, the adaptive changes that have comprised human evolution are, in a unified sense, both biological and social. Indeed, *biological is social* in this view (see Petersen & Taylor, 1980). Thus, Gould's ideas indicate that as a consequence of neoteny, humans' paedomorphosis has led to the emergence of great plasticity, plasticity that enables and results from the developing child's interactions with his or her familial and broader cultural context. Moreover, the link suggested by Gould between neoteny and the development of plasticity is supported by research indicating that neoteny has important implications for neuronal development.

For example, individual neurons develop highly specific synaptic connections during their ontogeny, and in the early stages of this ontogeny these connections are modifiable (Jacobson, 1969). This flexible period occurs at varying times for different types of neurons and, since human development is so strongly retarded, even mature adults retain significant plasticity. Additional evidence for the plasticity of adult neurons is found in the research reviewed by Cotman and Nieto-Sampedro (1982), by Greenough and Green (1981), and by Lynch and Gall (1979), discussed in Chapter 4; for example, the data reported by Greenough (e.g., 1975, 1978), also discussed in Chapter 4, provide morphological evidence for plasticity in the mature and aged human brain.

Having established the link between neoteny and plasticity, it becomes reasonable to predict that interventions aimed at modifying or enhancing brain organization and function may be appropriately administered in human developmental periods well beyond those of infancy and early childhood.

Microevolutionary and macroevolutionary change and the concept of exaptation

In Chapter 3 we reviewed some of the recent literature in molecular genetics. Included among the areas in molecular biology where rapid progress is being made were gene marking and mapping techniques, gene cloning, and in at least some cases gene therapy. To these we should now add the study of genome evolution. As noted by Schopf (1982, p. 438), there is a "relentless surge" in "molecular biology's incorporation of evolution into its . . . world" and a "continuing and growing quest for a material basis for genomic organization and genomic change, both in the development of individuals and in the origin of species.''

The scientific goal of those who study genome evolution – microevolutionary processes – is an ambitious one: to use knowledge gained from the study of molecular genetics to understand the relations among genomic processes, individual development (ontogeny), and the origin of species diversity – macroevolutionary change.

To illustrate the nature of this scientific agenda, note that while François Jacob (quoted in Lewin, 1982c, p. 718) indicates that ''the differences betwen adult organisms merely reflect differences in the developmental processes that produce them. . . . To really understand how evolution proceeds, it is necessary to understand embryological development and its limitations,'' understanding the presence or absence of such embryological developmental constraints involves understanding the associated links between micro- and macroevolutionary processes.

This role for this tripartite connection is indicated in the views of E. O. Wilson. To Wilson (in Lewin 1982d) the key concern in current evolutionary thinking involves the limits of the extent to which natural selection can provide a basis for historical plasticity in human processes. In other words, the key question is if natural selection is all-powerful:''Can it mold anything in an organism under the right circumstances? Or are there important constraints in the embryological development of organisms that proscribe the range of possibilities?'' (Quoted in Lewin, 1982d, p. 1092).

Lewontin (in Lewin, 1982c) agrees with Wilson that the answer to these questions lies in understanding the relation between molecular biology and traditional biology. Indeed, Lewontin contends that the central problem of evolution – the relation between microevolutionary change and macroevolutionary change – cannot be adequately addressed unless there is an integration of molecular and ''whole-animal'' biology.

But how can the study of genome evolution – which can be categorized into those investigations that focus largely on processes such as DNA transposition and gene amplification and those investigations that focus largely on products of these processes (e.g., transposable elements, highly repeated DNA, and moderately repeated DNA; Schopf, 1982) – be integrated with the study of macroevolutionary, whole-animal biology? And of what relevance is such an integration to understanding the potential plasticity of evolutionary processes?

The work of Gould and Vrba (1982) is relevant to these questions, for their work, in speaking to the relation between genome evolution and the origin of species diversity, offers a provocative new perspective about how evolutionary processes provide a basis for human plasticity.

To understand the potential of the contribution made by Gould and Vrba

(1982), it must be emphasized that their work deals with supplying a term to fill a conceptual lacuna in evolutionary biology. Gould and Vrba note that there are two current meanings in the biological literature for the term *adaptation*: First, "a feature is an adaptation only if it was built by natural selection for the function it now performs," whereas the second definition conceives of "adaptation in a static or immediate way as any feature that enhances current fitness, regardless of its historical origin" (p. 5).

To illustrate the use of these two distinct conceptions of the term, Gould and Vrba cite G. C. Williams (1966) as illustrating the first definition. Williams contended that one should speak of adaptation only when one can "attribute the origin and perfection of this design to a long period of selection for effectiveness in this particular role" (p. 6). Williams distinguishes further between adaptations and their functions (i.e., their operations), on the one hand, from fortuitous, "chance" effects, on the other. By *effect* Williams (1966) means simply something caused or produced (e.g., by a function), a result, or a consequence (e.g., of a function).

The writings of W. J. Bock (1967, 1979, 1980), in contrast to those of Williams, illustrate the second definition of adaptation. For instance, Bock (1979, p. 39) indicates that "an adaptation is . . . a feature of the organism . . . which interacts operationally with some factor of its environment so that the individual survives and reproduces."

Gould and Vrba (1982) believe that a confusion therefore exists about a concept central in evolutionary theory, a conflict arising as a consequence of "subsuming different criteria of historical genesis and current utility under a single term" (p. 5). Indeed, Darwin himself may have seen this potential confusion:

The sutures in the skulls of young mammals have been advanced as a beautiful adaptation for aiding paturition, and no doubt they facilitate, or may be indispensable for this act; but as sutures occur in the skulls of young birds and reptiles, which have only to escape from a broken egg, we may infer that this structure has arisen from the laws of growth, and has been taken advantage of in the parturition of the higher animals. (Darwin, 1859, p. 197)

In other words, while Darwin saw the necessity of unfused sutures in the skulls of young mammals, he eschewed – as Williams (1966) would argue later, one indeed should eschew – labeling the unfused sutures as adaptations. Darwin did this because the unfused sutures "were not built by selection to function as they now do in mammals" (Gould & Vrba, 1982). But if the unfused sutures are not adaptations, what are they? Clearly, the taxonomy of form in relation to fitness lacks a term, and this is the omission Gould and Vrba seek to rectify.

Following Williams (1966), they define

as an *adaptation* any feature that promotes fitness and was built by selection for its current role (criterion of *historical genesis*). The operation of an adaptation is its *function*. . . .

Table 2. *A taxonomy of fitness*

Process	Character		Usage
Natural selection shapes the character for a current-use – adaptation.	Adaptation		Function
A character, previously shaped by natural selection for a particular function (an adaptation), is coopted for a new use – cooptation.		Aptation	
A character whose origin cannot be ascribed to the direct action of natural selection (a nonaptation), is coopted for a current use – cooptation.	Exaptation		Effect

Source: Gould and Vrba (1982, p. 5).

We may also follow Williams in labelling the operation of a useful character not built by selection for its current role as an *effect*. (We designate as an effect only the usage of such a character, not the character itself . . .). . . . But what is the unselected, but useful character itself to be called? Indeed it has no recognized name. . . . Its space on the logical chart is currently blank.

We suggest that such characters, evolved for other usages (or for no function at all), and later "coopted" for their current role, be called *exaptations*. . . . They are fit for their current role, hence *aptus*, but they were not designed for it, and are therefore not *ad aptus*, or pushed towards fitness. They owe their fitness to features present for other reasons, and are therefore *fit (aptus) by reason of (ex)* their form, or *ex aptus*. Mammalian sutures are an exaptation for parturition. Adaptations have functions, exaptations have effects. The general, static phenomenon of being fit should be called aptation, not adaptation. (The set of aptations existing at any one time consists of two partially overlapping subsets: the subset of adaptations and the subset of exaptations. This also applies to the more inclusive set of aptations existing through time. (Gould & Vrba, 1982, p. 6)

The distinctions made by Gould and Vrba among adaptation, exaptation, and aptation are summarized in Table 2.

A clear implication of Gould and Vrba's revised terminology is that not all instances of fitness are adaptations; that is, not all features of an organism's structure and function that are aptational have this character as a consequence of being shaped by natural selection for this character. Such a possibility, if supported, would serve to weaken what Gould and Lewontin (1979) have labeled the "adaptationist program," the position that a feature's current aptational character implies historical shaping by natural selection for that character.

Lewontin (1981) has discussed the adaptationist "program" and its conventional use of the concept of adaptation. As do Gould and Vrba, Lewontin sees problems with the "adaptationist program" view of adaptation; in essence, he sees the view as deficient because it ignores the active, constructive role the organism plays in its own adaptation: It shapes the context to which it adapts, and hence the reciprocal, multilevel (i.e., dynamic interactional) relation between organism and context. In other words, Lewontin's criticisms of the conventional use of the concept of adaptation derive from a viewpoint consonant with the life-span probabilistic-epigenetic conception of development discussed in Chapters 1 and 2. Specifically, Lewontin (1981, p. 245) notes that biologists committed to the "adaptationist program"

define adaptation as "some kind of partial match with the external world." This is the view of a static, or at least independent, outer world that poses fixed problems to which the organism (or population) responds by fitting itself to the preexisting external condition.... But life is not like that. Organisms ... by their own life activities determine which aspects of the outer world make up their environment. Organisms change the environment by their activities. They transduce physical signals from the environment into new physical forms within themselves. Species do not, in general, "solve" preset environmental "problems" by gathering information and responding appropriately. Rather, they "construct" environments. The problem is that the concept of adaptation has been extended metaphorically from its valid domain of describing individual, short-term, goal-directed behavior to other levels. Individual organisms can be observed to be adaptive machines as they steer around obstacles, chase prey, defend themselves from attack, or push their roots around stones. But it is pure metaphor, ideologically molded by the progressivism and optimalism of the nineteenth century, to describe numbers of chromosomes, patterns of fertility, migrations, and religious institutions as "adaptations." It is this kind of error that led to the now discredited descriptions of lemming "migrations" and "mass suicides" as adaptive responses to crowding. It is not simply that some evolutionary process can be described as nonadaptive, but that the entire framework is in question. Whether we look at the fossil record or at living species, we do not see them as "adapting," but as "adapted." But how can that be? How is it that, if evolution is a process of *adapting*, organisms always seem to be *adapted*? It may be more illuminating to see organisms as *changing* and, in the process, as reconstructing the elements of the outer world into a new environment that is sufficient for their survival. To accept the metaphor of adaptation for human culture is to restrict the possible explanations of culture to a relatively narrow range. The price of metaphor is eternal vigilance.

Supporting the positions of Gould and Vrba (1982), Gould and Lewontin (1979) and Lewontin (1981) regarding the problems with the "adaptationist program" view of adaptation are data from microevolutionary research, which I will discuss below, which illustrate the potential role of exaptation in evolution (e.g., Doolittle & Sapienza, 1980; Orgel & Crick, 1980) and which further suggest that the basis for this microevolutionary exaptation lies in the possibility of there being substantial amounts of DNA that may be nonadaptive (or, better, nonaptative) at the level of the phenotype. Thus, Gould and Vrba (1982) contend that if nonaptation "is about to assume an important role in a revised evolutionary theory, then our terminology of form must recognize its cardinal evolutionary significance – cooptability for fitness" (p. 7). In other words, recognition of the potential presence of exaptative, aptative features leads one to recognize that previously nonaptative (note, *not* preadaptive) features may be present and may be coopted for fitness – a recognition that we will see provides a key for plasticity in evolutionary processes.

To indicate the precise bases of this contribution to plasticity, it is important to consider exaptation pertinent to the features of microevolution that we noted above. This illustration of exaptation indicates how this concept may account for a feature of the genome that, to those committed to an adaptationist program, might appear anomolous. Gould and Vrba (1982, p. 10) point out that

for a few years after Watson and Crick elucidated the structure of DNA, many evolutionists hoped that the architecture of genetic material might fit all their presuppositions about evolutionary processes. The linear order of nucleotides might be the beads on a string of classical genetics: one gene, one enzyme; one nucleotide substitution, one minute alteration for natural selection to scrutinize. We are now, not even 20 years later, faced with genes in pieces, complex hierarchies of regulation and, above all, vast amounts of repetitive DNA. High repetitive, or satellite, DNA can exist in millions of copies; middle-repetitive DNA, with its tens to hundreds of copies, forms about one quarter of the genome in both *Drosophilo* and *Homo*. What is all the repetitive DNA for (if anything)? How did it get there?

Some of the repeated DNA may be conventional adaptations, selected for a role in regulation (for example, the repeated copies may bring previously separated parts of the genome into new, aptative interrelation). However, there is too much repetitive DNA for such direct adaptation to account for all of it.

A second, traditional (i.e., adaptationist program-oriented) basis for the presence of so much repeated DNA has been forwarded. This suggestion is that repetitive DNA exists because it is needed for *future* evolution. That is, it exists to provide for a ''flexible future''; for instance, nonused, redundant copies are free to alter because their adaptative product is still being produced by the remaining DNA copies (e.g., Cohen, 1976; Kleckner, 1977). However, this second argument is teleological, in that it permits future needs to determine present circumstances.

While Gould and Vrba (1982) believe that future uses are quite significant consequences of repeated DNA, the potential future use cannot be held to empirically determine the prior status of the genome.

The concept of exaptation capitalizes on the idea that repeated DNA may indeed have a significant future use, but does so without recourse to teleological, ''final cause'' explanations. And in making these contributions, the concept of exaptation furthers understanding of how features of the genome provide a basis for plastic microevolutionary processes. Gould and Vrba (1982) explain that

defenders of the second tradition understand how important repetitive DNA is to evolution, but only know the conventional language of adaptation for expressing this conviction. But since utility is a future condition (when the redundant copy assumes a different function or undergoes secondary adaptation for a new role), an impasse in expression develops. To break this impasse, we might suggest that repeated copies are nonapted features, available for cooptation later, but not serving any direct function at the moment. When coopted, they will be exaptations in their new role (with secondary adaptive modifications if altered).

What then is the source of these exaptations? According to the first tradition, they arise as true adaptations and later assume their different function. The second tradition, we have argued, must be abandoned. A third possibility has recently been proposed (or, rather, better codified after previous hints): perhaps repeated copies can originate for no adaptive reason that concerns the traditional Darwinian level of phenotypic advantage (Orgel & Crick, 1980; Doolittle & Sapienza, 1980). Some DNA elements are transposable; if these can duplicate and move, what is to stop their accumulation as long as they remain invisible to the phenotype (if they become so numerous that they begin to exert energetic constraint upon the phenotype, then natural selection will eliminate them)? Such "selfish DNA" may be playing its own Darwinian game at a genic level, but it represents a true nonaptation at the level of the phenotype. Thus, repeated DNA may often arise as a nonaptation. Such a statement in no way argues against its vital importance for evolutionary futures. When used to great advantage in that future, these repeated copies are exaptations. (P. 11)

In other words, and crucial for the synthesis of micro- and macroevolutionary processes, Gould and Vrba (1982) believe that there exists an "enormous pool" of nonaptations and that this pool must be the source, the "reservoir," of most evolutionary flexibility. To again return to their words:

We need to recognize the central role of "cooptability for fitness" as the primary evolutionary significance of ubiquitous nonaptation in organisms. In this sense, and at its level of the phenotype, this nonaptive pool is an analog of mutation – a source of raw material for further selection.

Both adaptations and nonaptations, while they may have non-random approximate causes, can be regarded as randomly produced with respect to any potential cooptation by further regimes of selection. Simply put: all exaptations *originate* randomly with respect to their effects. Together, these two classes of characters, adaptations and nonaptations, provide an enormous pool of variability, at a level higher than mutations, for cooptation as exaptations [and provide for] ... the flexibility of phenotypic characters as a primary enhancer of or damper upon future evolutionary change. Flexibility lies in the pool of features available for cooptation (either as adaptations to something else that has ceased to be important in new selective regimes, as adaptations whose original function continues but which may be coopted for an additional role, or as nonaptations always potentially available). The paths of evolution – both the constraints and the opportunities – must be largely set by the size and nature of this pool of potential exaptations. Exaptive possibilities define the "internal" contribution that organisms make to their own evolutionary future. (Gould & Vrba, 1982, pp. 12, 13)

Conclusions

In sum, the concept of exaptation provides a potentially seminal contribution to modern evolutionary theory by virtue of its ability to address the key problem currently facing evolutionary biology, that of the relation between micro- and macroevolutionary processes. In addition to this potential benefit, the concept of exaptation leads to a further understanding of how the processes involved in evolution are plastic ones. Finally, the concept of exaptation is consistent with a theme presented throughout the book – that at the level of organism there exist processes that contribute to the organism's plasticity and that allow the organism to play a role in the development of its own flexibility. Organisms present to their context the exaptative possibilities that provide a key basis of their own future evolution.

In turn, and as noted in the first part of this chapter dealing with the implications of heterochrony in human evolution, Gould's ideas about the relation between neoteny and plasticity have relevance for areas of scholarship other than evolutionary biology. His work bears directly on comparative–developmental psychology and sociology's concern with the adaptive significance of individaul and group interdependencies and of intergenerational transmission. The next two chapters deal in turn with each of these areas.

7   Comparative-developmental psychological bases of plasticity

Perhaps more so than in any of the other disciplinary areas we have considered, the concept of "levels" and the idea that reciprocal interactions among levels provide a basis of processes' plasticity have played central roles in theory and research in comparative–developmental psychology. Moreover, while not as historically preeminent, the use of these notions specifically in the study of human ontogeny (i.e., in developmental psychology per se) is also quite important (see R. Lerner, 1976; R. Lerner & Busch-Rossnagel, 1981).

Psychological levels and functional orders

Interest in the nature of species evolutionary changes, in interspecies differences in species evolutionary changes, and in criteria for discriminating among species levels led evolutionary biologists and comparative psychologists to study the concept of *anagenesis* (Yarczower & Hazlett, 1977). Although a controversial idea (Capitanio & Leger, 1979; Yarczower & Hazlett, 1977; Yarczower & Yarczower, 1979), most scientists agree that "anagenesis refers to the evolution of increased complexity in some trait" (Capitanio & Leger, 1979, p. 876). For example, Dobzhansky et al. (1977, p. 236) note that "anagenetic episodes commonly create organisms with novel characters and abilities beyond those of their ancestors" or simply that anagenesis is an "evolutionary advance or change." Similarly, Jerison (1978, pp. 1–2) notes that an evolutionary analysis of progress from earlier to later species "is called 'anagenetic' and is about progressive evolution" and that in such an analysis "the objective is to identify grades in evolution." Thus, an anagenetic (evolutionary) advance would place a species at a different evolutionary grade (Gould, 1976), and location of a species at a different grade would mark interspecies differences in evolutionary changes, that is, anagenesis (Dobzhansky et al., 1977).

However, it is clear that an advance in complexity is often difficult to identify. For example, what specific structural and behavioral criteria need to be met (see Capitanio & Leger, 1979)? This is especially true when human psychosocial

105

behavior is involved (Yarczower & Hazlett, 1977; Yarczower & Yarczower, 1979). However, a useful framework is provided by Schneirla (1957, 1959, 1972; Tobach & Schneirla, 1968; see also, e.g., Birch & Lefford, 1963; Tobach, 1978; Sherrington, 1951).

Schneirla (1972, p. 200) noted that "the principle of levels has come into current usage through a recognition of important differences in the complexity, the degree of development, and the interdependent organization of behavior functions throughout the animal series." As did Huxley (1958), Schneirla recognized that "adaptivity" is a characteristic of all extant levels of organization and could not be used in and of itself as a criterion to differentiate among levels (see too Yarczower & Hazlett, 1977). Accordingly, to differentiate among levels, Schneirla (1972, p. 231) argued that

the levels considered lowest are those on which specific biological processes account directly for the character of adaptive behavior, without further hierarchies of complexity in the organization; the progressively higher levels are marked by the presence of progressive linked stages of organization typified by increased qualitative complexity in perception and learning; the highest levels are those of plastic adaptive adjustments arising through widened learning capacities and the entrance of thinking.

Schneirla (1957) proposes the use of a behavioral *stereotypy–plasticity continuum* in order to differentiate the levels of complexity representative of different species. Stereotyped behavior shows a high correspondence between sensory input and motor output. It is "sense-dominated" behavior (Hebb, 1949). There is little intraindividual change across time within situations. Plastic behavior – or, in the terms presented in Chapter 1, flexible behavior – shows considerable response variability given invariant sensory input. There is intraindividual change across time within situations. Moreover, Schneirla indicates that this continuum must be understood along with two other key concepts: *psychological levels* and *functional orders*.

Organisms at higher psychological levels are those whose most ontogenetically advanced level of functioning shows considerable plasticity (i.e., flexibility in the behavioral repertoire). Their initial ontogenetic periods will show "sense-dominated" behavior. However, after a relatively long developmental period in comparison to organisms more stereotyped in their final functional level (Hebb, 1949; Schneirla, 1957), they will progress to this plastic level. These characteristics of progression through their functional order are based on the greater ratio of association to sensory fibers (A/S ratio; Hebb, 1949) representative of the psychological level (Thompson, 1981).

Thus, in organisms with higher A/S ratios a longer time is necessarily involved in the organization of this structure (R. Lerner, 1976). In turn, however, organisms at lower psychological levels are those whose functional order is characterized by a more stereotyped final form. However, presumably because they have less structure to organize (have a lower A/S ratio), they reach this last point in their functional order relatively sooner in their ontogeny than do organisms at higher psychological levels (R. Lerner, 1976).

We see here then that Schneirla (1957) reaches a conclusion from his knowledge of the comparative–developmental literature that, in the previous chapter of this book, we have seen Gould (1977) reach in his review of the evolutionary biology literature. That is, the key difference between humans and animals at other (lower) psychological levels is a neotenous one. Indeed, this role of human neoteny in accounting for both physical and cognitive–behavioral differences between humans and other species is so strongly established that scientists who on other matters hold widely divergent views, for example, Schneirla (1957) and Lorenz (1965), agree on this point (e.g., see Lorenz, 1971).

Thus, although Gould (1977) notes that the correlation across the animal series of maturation with loss of both cognitive/behavioral and physical plasticity is well established, because of neoteny the relation does not hold for humans. Their neoteny "postpones," or even circumvents, the link between completion of maturation and loss of plasticity, and is the precise reason why they "reach higher levels of organization" (Gould, 1977, p. 401).

Moreover, it is Lorenz (1971) who has paid particular attention to the import of human neoteny for the presence and development of behavioral flexibility. Lorenz has repeatedly emphasized the "juvenile" (paedomorphic) character of human behavioral plasticity. He asks, "What is the source of this remarkable persistent juvenile characteristic of investigative curiosity in human beings, which is so fundamental to the essence of humanity?" (p. 279). His answer is that "the constructive character of man – the maintenance of active, creative interaction with the environment – is a neotenous phenomenon" (p. 180) and that "human exploratory inquisitive behavior – restricted in animals to a brief developmental phase – is extended to persist until the onset of senility" (p. 239). In other words, Lorenz (1971), like Gould (1977), sees neoteny as providing the basis of human plasticity – and, also like Gould (1977), he sees such plasticity as arising as a consequence of humans' interactions with their context. Finally, like Gould (1977), Cotman and Nieto-Sampedro (1982), Greenough and Green (1981), Jacobson (1969), and Lynch and Gall (1979), Lorenz sees the potential for such plasticity as existing across the life span.

Thus, in converging with data from both evolutionary biology and comparative–developmental psychology, Schneirla's (1957, 1959) ideas have relevance for both the phylogenetic and the ontogenetic changes of humans. Human evolution should be characterizable by progressively greater potentials for flexibility – to change and to adapt to change. Huxley (1958, p. 452) agrees. He notes that

adaptation is not merely the capacity to survive, nor is it merely to the immediate present. It also covers adaptation to change; and when change is so rapid and drastic as it can be in the psychosocial sector, adaptation to change and to the direction of change may become of overriding importance.

Quite consistent with the theme I have been developing throughout this book, then, is the view of Schneirla (1957, 1959, 1972) and of Huxley (1958) that human plasticity not only represents the *potential* for intraindividual change, but more importantly the *capacity* to show (the actuality of) flexibility in the face of contextual – and perhaps, particularly psychosocial – presses. Thus, flexibility becomes a key feature of human adaptation, one arising from the interaction of the plastic processes at the constituent levels of analysis comprising the human condition. Such multilevel plasticity of process provides then a rich matrix of covariation for intervention; because of the embeddedness of the individual in his or her context, a vast array of techniques may be used to optimize human life.

However, it should be reemphasized that although evolution has led to the presence of our potential for plasticity, its basis, in structure, requires organization over the course of ontogeny. As such, normative patterns of human ontogeny should be characterizable by the progressively greater presence of plasticity. There are data supporting these ideas.

In evolutionary biology, Lewontin and Levins (1978) provide evidence for the link between anagenesis, complexity, plasticity, and what they term "coupling–uncoupling" phenomena. Lewontin and Levins (1978, p. 79) cite Hegel's warning "that the organism is made up of arms, legs, head and trunk only as it passes under the knife of the anatomist," and note that "the intricate interdependence of the parts of the body ... permit survival when they function well, but in pathological conditions produce pervasive disaster." However, such interdependence of parts is neither phylogenetically nor ontogenetically static. Relations among parts change over the course of evolution; often this involves the rapid evolution of some characteristics, or "traits," and the relative constancy of others. In other words, while various aspects of an organism may be bound together as "traits" if they are either units of development or selection, they may lose their cohesion and evolve independently if the direction of selection is altered (Lewontin & Levins, 1978).

Indeed, there are several aspects of adaptation that suggest that tight integration of "traits," or in Lewontin and Levins' terms, coupling, is disadvantageous. First, a given characteristic may be subject to alternative selection pressures. If the optimal states of the characteristics under the separate pressures are not vastly different, then adaptation would be best served by a "compromise in which the part in question is determined by" all the presses. Second, the uncoupling of "traits" is advantageous "as the number of interacting variables and the intensity of their interaction increases (Lewontin & Levins, 1978, pp. 84 – 4); this is the case because in the face of these increases it becomes increasingly difficult for selective pressures to increase fitness. Thus, species with very tight coupling will be unable to adapt as readily as those in which the different components which increase fitness are more autonomous. Third, the more strongly coupled and interdependent the "traits" of an organism are, the more pervasive is the damage done to an organism when some stressor overwhelms a particular "trait."

Accordingly, what has occurred over the course of evolution is that the advantages of coordinated functioning and mutual regulation have come to oppose the disadvantages of excessive constraint and hence vulnerability and that, at least at the human level, organisms may have the capacity to successively couple and uncouple "traits." Ontogenetically then, it may be that the most adaptive organisms are those that have the potential to develop the capacity to couple and uncouple traits as the context demands – for example, to show flexibility in the organization of their behavioral repertoire in order to fit the demands of their context (Lerner & Lerner, 1983). We may suggest then that the direction of evolution at the human level has been to move toward providing the substrate for the coupling–uncoupling of "traits." This is what may be involved in anagenesis. That is, if higher evolutionary grades are defined as being more complex and if greater complexity means greater plasticity, a key instance of such plastic processes would be the capability to couple, uncouple, and couple anew – either through recoupling or with ontogenetically unique couplings. This facility should become progressively established across ontogeny, as the physiological substrate of the psychological level of analysis becomes organized.

In sum, although plasticity is a key component of adaptation across the animal series (Huxley, 1958), animals at different psychological levels may be distinguished on the basis of the final level of plasticity they attain across their ontogeny (Schneirla, 1957, 1972). Thus, plastic functioning that both derives from and enables the organism's interactions with (embeddedness in) its context must be understood as a developmental phenomenon. The several points involved in this position are supported by data from both comparative and developmental psychological research.

Plasticity: comparative and developmental bases

Plasticity at different psychological levels

Although animals differ in the final level of plasticity reached across their life span and in the time it takes to reach that level, there is evidence that across the animal series plasticity exists and subserves adaptation (Huxley, 1958). The capability of organisms of a specific genotype to express alternative morphotypes in different ecological conditions is termed *developmental polymorphism* (Gilbert, 1980); this concept is related to the "norm of reaction" notion (Hirsch,

1970), which indicates that any one genotype can, in interaction with different environments, lead to different phenotypes. Both concepts underscore the plastic nature of the relation between genes and developmental outcomes and the role of the context in moderating this relation. Comparative analysis of the development of various species of protozoans and invertebrates indicates that the environment in which an individual develops can greatly affect both its size and its shape (Gilbert, 1980), as well as its individual and social behavior.

For example, such developmental polymorphism has been identified in many insects. Adult aphids develop wings only when the host plants on which they feed become unsuitable and movement to new plants thus becomes advantageous (Gilbert, 1980). Both crowding from other individuals on the inadequate host plant (and the physical stimulation this crowding provides) and the poor nutritional level of the inadequate host plant affect the endocrine system of the aphid larvae and induce the development of a winged adult. These observations illustrate the link between plasticity and adaptation I have been emphasizing.

Other illustrations exist. Among protozoans, it is known that when the *Tetrahymena vorax* feeds on bacteria or assimilates organic compounds it reaches a length of 30–100 μm and has a small mouth; but when it feeds on other ciliated protozoans, it has an exceedingly large mouth and a length of 150–200 μm (Gilbert, 1980). Similarly, in some species of the crustacean water flea *Daphnia*, embryos develop into individuals with large and helmeted heads only when the water becomes warm, turbulent, and plentiful with food (Gilbert, 1980).

Another example of developmental polymorphism and plasticity among organisms of relatively minimal complexity is provided by the rotifer *Asplanchna*. Rotifers are metazoans, 50–2,000 μm long, and comprised of about 1,000 cells. In level of complexity they are approximately between flatworms (e.g., *Planaria*) and roundworms (*Ascaris*), and they are found commonly in ponds and lakes (Gilbert, 1980). Gilbert finds that in several species of *Asplanchna* (e.g., *A. Sieboldi*) three different female morphotypes can be expressed by individuals derived parthenogenetically from a single female (and hence having the same exact genes). Gilbert finds that the control of morphotype expression is completely attributable to the influence of environmental factors during development – specifically, the level of dietary vitamin E. These differences are in size, shape, and, most interestingly, in behavior (e.g., likelihood to be cannibalistic) and physiology (e.g., modes of reproduction). Developmental polymorphism in the *Asplanchna* allows the organism to adapt rapidly to changing ecological conditions.

Moreover, as Hutchinson (1981) points out, the illustration of *Asplanchna* is not unique in the animal series. She indicates that "throughout the living world there are many polymorphic species in which the polymorphism persists because the characters of a particular morph, though rarely useful and in fact slightly detrimental most of the time, are of extraordinary value when the morph is at all favored" (p. 161).

As evidenced by Gilbert's (1980) work with the *Asplanchna*, the plasticity involved in developmental polymorphism in organisms of low levels of complexity extends to features of their behavior. Such behavioral plasticity in organisms of low complexity levels is also illustrated in work reported by Fox and Morrow (1981) on feeding specialization in herbivorous insects. They report that although many herbivorous insects have generalized diets over the particular specie's entire geographical range, it is incorrect to assume that diet breadth is a fixed species characteristic. Rather, Fox and Morrow report, these insects function as specialists with restricted diets in local communities and that, within overall phylogenetic constraints, specialization is often a plastic attribute of a population that is adapting to social and ecological features of its particular community.

Other research involving insects suggests that their social behavior is affected by context (Uetz, Kane, & Stratton, 1982) and that insect reproductive behavior may involve learning (Prokopy et al., 1982). Uetz et al. (1982), for example, report that in response to climate and to availability of prey, the spider *Metepeira spinipes* varies in group size – from solitary existence to living in aggregations of from 5 to 150 or more individuals – and in interindividual distance within the colony. Prokopy et al. (1982) have found evidence of associative learning in apple maggot flies. Learning during oviposition in apple hosts may significantly influence the probability of these insects accepting or rejecting these hosts in future encounters.

As a final example of the presence of a mechanism providing the potential for flexibility within a relatively uncomplex organism, we may note Dyer and Gould's (1981) findings regarding honeybees' ability on cloudy days to navigate to familiar food sources and orient their dances accurately. This navigational backup system was found to be based on the bees' memory of the diurnal course of the sun with respect to local landmarks – as opposed to a more reflexive, magnetic compass sense, an ability to perceive the sun, or patterns of polarized light through the clouds.

Of course, species of greater complexity than protozoans and invertebrates also show plastic processes across their development. In some species of birds, for example, reproductive output shows flexibility in response to contextual influences. Högstedt (1980) finds that among territorial birds, like magpies, which have to forage for their food, reproductive output (e.g., from enlarged to reduced broods) varies optimally in relation to differences in the quality of foraging territories; about 85% of the within-years variation in clutch size was associated with such differences between territories. Moreover, colonial bird species, which lack individual foraging areas, have a smaller clutch size than territorial species.

Still other illustrations of the presence of plasticity across the animal series include plasticity of social organizational processes among insects (e.g., army ants; Schneirla, 1957, 1959; Tobach & Schneirla, 1968), birds, and other relatively uncomplex mammals. Recent research by Stacey and Bock (1978), for example, indicates that acorn woodpeckers in southeastern Arizona exhibit two quite different types of social organization, one involving high cooperation and the establishment of resident groups, the other migration and only temporary formation (during reproduction) of male–female pairs. That both patterns occur in the same population suggests a high degree of social plasticity in this species (Stacey & Bock, 1978).

In regard to some specific individual and social behaviors, we may note that recognition of and aggression toward enemies are also flexible features of many animals' behavioral repertoire. Moreover, there is evidence that in many species this flexibility involves observational learning and imitation processes. Curio, Ernst, and Vieth (1978), for example, found evidence for the social transmission of enemy recognition and of aggressive (mobbing) acts toward the enemy in birds. Using captive European blackbirds as subjects, these authors allowed a subject to witness a conspecific mob a novel but harmless bird (an Australian honeyeater). This bird was chosen as the conditioned stimulus because, although it is of a size similar to some of blackbirds' predators, it is both novel and in details other than size resembles no genuine predator. As a consequence of their observation experience the blackbirds imitated their "teacher," or model, and mobbed the honeyeater, both when the model was present and when it was absent. Moreover, the mobbing response persisted during subsequent presentations of the novel bird alone; and the novel bird remained a more effective conditioned stimulus than an artificial control object.

In addition, Curio et al. report that the imitating birds could be used as teachers for other birds: enemy recognition and mobbing could be transmitted along a chain of at least six individuals. Curio et al. interpret this last finding as evidence supporting the possibility of cultural transmission among birds. That is, plasticity in part involves varying one's behavioral repertoire to meet (adapt to) potentially unique contextual presses. If these adaptations remain useful, so that they continue to play a role, for example, among younger generations, then it would be particularly useful if they could be interindividually transmitted. When a species evolves the capacity for observational learning and imitation, one mechanism for such interindividual influence has been established. Thus, while the results of Curio et al. are provocative in suggesting the presence of these processes in birds, they are also quite important in that they allow us to see the links among adaptation and plastic processes (here observational learning and imitative learning ones), on the one hand, and among adaptation, plastic processes, and intergenerational transmission, on the other. The former links are already the subject of a rich literature in regard to both research and intervention in human development (e.g., Bandura, 1965, 1971, 1977, 1980a, b; Kendall, 1981; Kendall & Hollon, 1979). In fact, according to Hutchinson (1981), imitation has played a key role, to date unappreciated, in human adaptation and evolution. The latter links will, in Chapters 8 and 9, also be evaluated for their implications for research and intervention. Here, however, we may note one other illustration of the plasticity of social organization processes that exists in even relatively uncomplex mammalian species.

Hoogland (1982) found that black-tailed prairie dogs have a repertoire of several behavioral mechanisms by which they can avoid inbreeding. Hoogland observed a colony of these animals for six years and discovered that the colony is composed of contiguous but separate family groups (coteries). The animals within any coterie almost never mated with close genetic relatives. Such inbreeding was avoided by (1) a male leaving his natal coterie before breeding, thus leaving his female relatives behind; (2) an adult male leaving the coterie before his daughters matured; (3) a young female being less likely to come into estrus if her father is in her coterie; and (4) an estrous female behaviorally avoiding mating with a father, a son, or a brother in her coterie. Thus, in their natural habitat this species of prairie dog shows evidence for plastic social organization processes, processes which give the animal considerable flexibility – in this case, several means by which mating with genetically close relatives is avoided.

In sum, consistent with the views of Schneirla (1957, 1972) and Huxley (1958), there is evidence that across the animal series plasticity is a key contributor to adaptation. A second key component of their views is that this plasticity involves the embeddedness of the organism in its context: The biological processes that enable plastic psychosocial functioning are themselves modified by this functioning. There are data in support of this idea as well.

Contextual influences on biological functioning

In my preceding discussions of the nature and implications of plasticity at several levels of analysis – for example, as uncovered by research on gene mapping, on recombinant DNA techniques, on neuroanatomy, and on neurochemistry and neurotransmitters – several instances were given of bidirectional influences among biological and psychosocial variables. Within the literature of comparative–developmental psychology other instances exist. Examples may be drawn from work done on prenatal and perinatal periods, as well as from postnatal periods extending through to adolescence.

For example, indicative of the idea that even the unborn organism is embedded in a social context is the fact that the embryonic and fetal development of many species of animals, including humans, can be influenced by the experiences, biochemistry, and drug and alcohol intake of the mother (see, e.g., Streissguth et al., 1980). For instance, Jonakait, Bohn, and Black (1980) report that the maternal experiences of pregnant rats, specifically in regard to treatment involving different levels of reserpine, had effects on the neurons of the developing embryos; and Woolf, Bixby, and Capranica (1976) report that a single two-hour exposure to auditory stimulation at any point during the final three days of incubation of Japanese quail accelerates their hatching. This three-day period includes both prenatal and perinatal stages of incubation, and these results suggest that the avian embryo is an entity responsive to sensory stimulation, as may for example be provided by the mother or other conspecifics.

Another, quite interesting example of the potential role of the prenatal social context is provided by the work of Meisel and Ward (1981). These researchers note that the capacity of normal female rats to exhibit male sexual behaviors (e.g., the motor pattern of ejaculating males, malelike mounting patterns) apparently depends on prenatal exposure to androgen, since such behaviors are reduced markedly by prenatal treatment with antiandrogenic drugs. However, the mechanism by which this exposure to androgen occurred remained unclear until Meisel and Ward determined that female rats are masculinized in utero by male littermates sharing the same uterine horn; specifically, females were found to be masculinized by the presence of males on the caudal side of the females. Since uterine blood flow in the rat is from the direction of the cervix toward the ovary, masculinizing hormones secreted by fetal males appear to be carried via the uterine vasculature to female littermates located downstream. Thus, the physical location of males sharing the same uterine space influences the later life (adult) sexual behaviors of female rats.

There is other evidence that features of the prenatal context can affect adult behavior in several species. Abel, Bush, and Dintcheff (1981) administered alcohol to pregnant rats twice daily throughout gestation. At birth, the offspring were tested for their thermogenic responsiveness to various drugs and to cold. Abel et al. found that prenatal exposure to alcohol resulted in tolerance to alcohol and cross-tolerance to pentobarbital and diazepam, but did not result in cross-tolerance to chlorpromazine, morphine, and d-amphetamine and did not affect responsiveness to cold. They interpret this pattern of effects as suggesting that prenatal exposure to alcohol produces specific long-term effects on the neural mechanisms underlying drug tolerance. Moreover, they report that adult learning deficits exist in rats treated prenatally with alcohol, suggesting that a prenatal contextual influence can have effects at multiple levels – here physiological and cognitive–behavioral – that may be potentially long-term.

Support for the finding of Abel et al. (1981) that chemicals in the prenatal context can have long-term effects on cognitive–behavioral functions is provided by the research of Bertolini and Poggioli (1981). Rats were treated with chloramphenicol – a broad-spectrum antibiotic widely used in Europe and many Latin countries – from days 7 to 21 of intrauterine life or in the first 3 days of extrauterine life. The rats were trained for avoidance conditioning when they were 60 days old. In all treated groups response acquisition was impaired to a highly significant degree.

The human fetus is, as noted above, also susceptible to prenatal influences. However, the multiple levels of the context within which even the unborn human is embedded often provide for more subtle and complex contextual influences. A study by Peters, Preston-Martin, and Yu (1981) illustrates this complexity by indicating that parental occupational role may eventuate in disease-producing agents being introduced to the fetus and that this introduction may come through the father or the mother. Peters et al. selected 92 cases of brain tumor in children less than 10 years old and compared these cases with 92 matched controls for parental occupational history. The cases were more likely than controls to show maternal occupations involving chemical exposure, paternal occupations involving solvents, and employment of father in the aircraft industry. These three factors were not affected by adjustment for the potential confounding variables examined (e.g., patterns of food consumption, drug use, alcohol use, and smoking habits). The authors note that while the mechanism of maternal influence is evident and akin to that associated with the introduction to the fetus of other teratogenic agents by the mother, the mechanisms of paternal influence are more subtle and less well documented. Such influence could be transmitted genetically, at conception, or in turn teratogens in the father's semen could affect the fetus after conception (e.g., see Kolata, 1978). In addition, teratogens from the soiled clothes of the father could be one of many other paternal sources of influences.

Regarding prenatal contextual influences, then, the above data indicate that the in utero organism is responsive to both proximal and distal contextual influences. Most of the examples of this sensitivity, however, illustrate that the context may have a deleterious effect on the prenatal organism. Two points are useful to note here. First, as emphasized in Chapter 1, the plasticity that provides us with the potential for change represents a "double-edged sword." We cannot be both capable of change and impervious to contextual sources of change that may result in undesirable outcomes. The presence of plasticity has both positive, potentially adaptive features and, in turn, limitations. The presence of plasticity means that we have the potential for successful intervention, but it also means that planned and unplanned interventions may have undesired direct and indirect effects. Of course, what is desirable to one person may be undesirable to another. The issue here is one of values and, as also suggested in Chapter 1, one cannot avoid confronting the issue of values in intervention. Indeed, I will return to this issue, as well as the issue of the limitations of plasticity, in the last chapter of this book. Here, however, it is useful to leave the topic of prenatal contextual influences, and of the issues this topic has allowed us to raise, and turn to further illustrations of the role of contextual influences in periods of life following the prenatal one.

Experiences in infancy also influence biological development. For example, a simple avoidance training procedure during early development has been found to produce massive neural traces in the visual and somatic cortices of kittens reared in a normal environment (Spinelli & Jensen, 1979). For instance, a preponderance of cells in these cortical areas had later response "preferences" for the stimuli used during training, and some of these cells exhibited properties not found in normal animals not receiving such training. As did the data reviewed by Cotman and Nieto-Sampedro (1982) and by Greenough and Green (1981), the Spinelli and Jensen data suggest that even in a normal environment there are potential influences that can substantially alter brain development. Combined with the findings we have already reviewed in Chapter 4 on the effects of environmental deprivation and enrichment on brain structure (e.g., recall the results of Greenough and colleagues – Greenough, 1975, 1978; Greenough & Green, 1981), the results of Spinelli and Jensen suggest that the development of the brain is responsive to both typical and atypical features of the organism's social context.

The role of the context within which organisms develop is of course not limited to physical–environmental influences. Feener (1981) provides an example of the often subtle yet crucial (for survival) social influences of the context on insect behavior patterns. Feener found that the parasitic phorid fly *Apocephalus* shifts the competitive balance between the ant species *Pheidole dentata* and *Solenopsis texana* by interfering with the defensive behavior of *P. dentata* major workers or soldiers.

The impact of the social context on biological development also may be shown during primate adolescence. Coe, Levine, and their colleagues (e.g., Coe & Levine, 1981; Coe et al.,1981) conducted a series of studies on the links between hormonal changes at puberty and psychosocial experiences in squirrel monkeys. Generally, their results indicate that the endocrine system at this time of life responds "not only to stressful events, but also to psychosocial factors such as the presence of opposite-sex partners or position in the social hierarchy" (Coe & Levine, 1981, pp. 14–15). In addition, the data of Coe et al. (1981) suggest that social facilitation may be extremely important for the coordination of reproductive cycles; longitudinal assessments of plasma progesterone levels indicated that the onset of ovarian cycles tended to be synchronized among females.

Similarly, there are data indicating that the contribution of hormones to monkey sexual behavior is moderated by the physical features of the context within which the hormone–behavior relation exists. While among humans it would come as little surprise to find that features of the physical setting can inhibit sexual activity, it has recently been reported that rhesus monkeys also show such responsivity to their context. Wallen (1982) observed the sexual behavior of rhesus monkeys in 15 male–female pairings in both a large and a small area during the follicular and luteal phases of the female's cycle. In all tests at the follicular phase, and in 53% of tests at the luteal phase, males ejaculated. However, in the large area, but not in the small one, a significant decline in ejaculation occurred during the luteal phase. Wallen concludes that the degree to which the rhesus pairs' sexual behavior was influenced by the female's hormonal state depended on the spatial conditions wherein the sexual behavior occurred.

Moreover, given the greater plasticity of higher psychological levels – as evidenced, say, by the use of cognitive, behavioral, and interpersonal processes in the control of human biological processes (as illustrated by the behavioral and cognitive–behavioral therapeutic techniques to control hypertension; see Holroyd, Appel, & Andrasik, in press, for a review of such interventions) – we might expect that at the human psychological level contextual (e.g., psychosocial) variables might play even a greater role than they do in squirrel or rhesus monkeys in moderating the impact of pubertal hormonal changes and of hormone–behavior relations. Such an inference is consistent with data reported by McClintock (1971, 1981). McClintock (1981) notes that complex social signals among groups of human females can either enhance or suppress ovarian cyclicity. An earlier study by McClintock (1971) illustrates the complex social embeddedness of the human female's menstrual cycle. McClintock studied 135 female residents of a college dormitory aged 17 to 22 years. Three times during the academic year, McClintock asked each subject when her last and second to last menstrual periods had begun, thus determining the date of onset for all cycles between late September and early April of the school year. McClintock found that there was a significant increase in synchronization – defined by her as a decrease in the difference between onset dates – among roommates and among closest friends. Furthermore, she determined that the significant factor in synchrony was that the individuals of the group spent time together.

Thus, social variables appear to exert a great influence in humans on what may ordinarily be thought of as a purely biological process. Data indicating that human adolescent behavior presumably linked to biological processes is greatly influenced by social influences is provided by Dornbusch et al. (1981). These researchers assessed the link between level of sexual maturation and the social behavior of dating among more than 7,000 12- to 17-year-old adolescents. Individual levels or rates of sexual maturation did not account for large proportions of the variance in dating (after age had been taken into account). Instead, it appeared that social pressures, involving behavior considered appropriate at a particular age, were the major determinant of onset of dating in adolescents. Dornbusch et al. conclude that their data illustrate that contextual influences such as social standards can reduce significantly the impact of an individual's biological processes on his or her behavior. In turn, other human biological processes associated with puberty – for example, those involved in menarche – appear to show a "secular trend" (Garn, 1980; Katchadourian, 1977); that is, they seem to be moderated by sociocultural variables that change across history (although there is some controversy surrounding the precise parameters of the historical change; Bullough, 1981; Eveleth & Tanner, 1976).

Finally, it should be noted that the comparative–developmental literature provides numerous instances of the role of psychosocial factors in the development of biological disorders. Two recent examples suffice not only to illustrate this link but, more importantly, to suggest the use of multidisciplinary research and intervention. Data reported by Sklar and Anisman (1979) suggest that stress can enhance tumor growth. A single session of inescapable shock administered to male mice resulted in earlier tumor appearance (of syngeneic P815 mastocytoma), exaggeration of tumor size, and decreased survival time. However, escapable shock had no such effects, and if mice were given long-term shock treatment (i.e., therapy in "coping"), then the effects of the inescapable shock were mitigated.

Similarly, the results of a study of Nerem, Levesque, and Cornhill (1980) indicate that it is possible to intervene, through psychosocial means, to ameliorate or even prevent biological disorders. Rabbits on a 2% cholesterol diet were individually petted, held, talked to, and played with on a regular basis. Examination at the end of the experimental period, including measurement of serum cholesterol levels, heart rate, and blood pressure, revealed that experimental animals showed more than 60% less aortic surface exhibiting sudanophilic lesions compared to controls (given the same diet and normal laboratory animal care) – even though serum cholesterol levels, heart rate, and blood pressure were comparable. In other words, the psychosocial context of the experimental group of rabbits served as an effective intervention technique in the prevention or diminution of aortic lesions.

The data of both Nerem et al. (1980) and Sklar and Anisman (1979) illustrate that variables in the psychological and social context of organisms not only affect the presence and development of biological disorders but also that the psychosocial context can be exploited as an effective source of interventions. These data underscore the role that psychologists trained in behavioral and/or cognitive behavioral individual interventions as well as social and community psychologists and sociologists trained in interventions with groups and institutions can play in collaborations with biologists and physicians. In sum, the ideas of Schneirla (1957, 1959, 1972) on the interrelation of biological, psychological, and social levels of analysis in animal behavior and development find support in the comparative–developmental literature, and as such have important implications for multidisciplinary research and intervention. Similarly, as we now turn to the final key idea that Schneirla forwards in regard to the role of plasticity in development – that plasticity must be understood as a developmental phenomenon – we also find support in the comparative–developmental literature.

Plasticity as a developmental phenomenon

In Schneirla's (1957) view, both evolutionary and ontogenetic progression involve progressive change toward greater plasticity of functioning. The view that such progressions occur across the animal series and, in particular, characterize the human psychological level is supported by several lines of evidence.

Birch and Lefford (1963, p. 3) note that the essential evolutionary strategy in the emergence of the mammalian nervous system from lower forms "has been the development of mechanisms for improved interaction among the separate sensory modalities." In turn, currently evolved organisms can be differentiated on the basis of their structural capability for plasticity at their highest functional order. They note that "as one ascends in the vertebrate series from fish to man the unimodal sensory control of behavior comes to be superseded by multimodal and intersensory control mechanisms" (p. 3). Similarly, Sherrington (1951, pp. 187–289) indicated that

the naive would have expected evolution in its course to have supplied us with more various sense organs for ampler perception of the world.... The policy has rather been to bring by the nervous system the so-called "five" into closer touch with one another.... A central clearing house of sense has grown up.... Not new senses, but better liaison between old senses is what the developing nervous system has in this respect stood for.

In turn, in regard to human ontogeny, Schneirla's (1957) ideas find support in Birch and Lefford's (1963) study of intersensory integration in 5- to 11-year-old children. Information received by the children through one sense modality (visual, haptic, or kinesthetic) was not directly transduced to another at all age levels. Rather, intersensory integrative ability showed a negatively accelerated increase across this age span, indicating that the presence of intermodal equivalence is a developmental phenomenon. Abravanel (1968) not only replicated these findings with children ranging in age from 3.3 years to 14.2 years, but found that covarying with these increments in perceptual plasticity was an increase in the child's activity in exploration of the stimulus. In addition, more differentiated motor behavior developed as fine finger movements replaced the use of the less effective palms.

The role played here by the organism's own activity in the development of its own plasticity has been identified in other human data sets reported by Piaget (1961; Piaget & Inhelder, 1956) and by Birch and Lefford (1967). In addition, experimental research with animals (Held & Hein, 1963) confirms this role of the organism's activity. Littermate kittens were or were not allowed to make motor adjustments as they traversed a circular route. Those animals making the active motor adjustments later performed better on a visual cliff apparatus than did the restricted animals.

All the above lends empirical support to the idea, advanced by Schneirla (1957), as well as by Hebb (1949), Piaget (1961; Piaget & Inhelder, 1956), Bühler (1928), and Baldwin (1897) that human plasticity is a developmental phenomenon, as well as support for the notion that the organism itself actively provides a basis of this progression. Numerous additional data sets indicate how children and adolescents, through their physical and behavioral characteristics of individuality, are producers of their development and how useful interventions may be built as a consequence of such "child effects" (R. Lerner, 1982; R. Lerner & Busch-Rossnagel, 1981). Here, however, it may suffice to indicate that the link between the child's own activity and perceptual development allows us to suggest one potential arena for intervention, one illustrating the potential role of the active individual.

Sex differences in spatial cognition and perception are among the best-documented ones in the developmental literature (Liben, Patterson, & Newcomb, 1981; Wittig & Petersen, 1979). Explanations of these differences range from those stressing native neurohormonal mechanisms to those emphasizing socialization differences (Wittig & Petersen, 1979). Whether or not differential histories of active, organized exploratory activities characterize male and female children manifesting the typical sex-specific behaviors, an intervention involving a change in previously existing behaviors to ones more active and differentiated might enhance cognitive/perceptual performance. That is, enhancing the child's active motor exploration of a stimulus might facilitate the child's perceptual development.

Conclusions

Work consistent with Schneirla's ideas suggests that interactions among the levels of analysis that comprise organisms and their contexts provide a basis of plasticity. The individual's developing plasticity both derives from and contributes to these interactions, and such contributions suggest the centrality of the individual's own activity in his or her own development. As such, research concerned with describing and/or facilitating the development of the individual's sense of self (e.g., Lewis & Brooks-Gunn, 1979) and self-regulatory behaviors and cognitions (Kendall, 1981; Kendall & Hollon, 1979) should contribute immeasurably to enhancing the repertoire of useful interventions.

Indeed, there are animal data supportive of this point. Visintainer, Volpicelli, and Seligman (1982) have demonstrated that the expression of self-regulatory behavior can significantly influence an organism's rejection of cancer and enhance its survival. These authors implanted tumors in rats who, one day later, experienced inescapable, escapable, or no electric shock. They report that while only 27% of the rats receiving inescapable shock rejected the tumor, 63% of the rats who received escapable shock rejected the tumor; among the rats who experienced no shock, 54% rejected the tumor. Visintainer et al. conclude that an organism's lack of control over stressors reduces tumor rejection and decreases survival, while, conversely, control over stressors increases tumor rejection and survival. If results like this are replicated among humans, then behavioral and cognitive behavioral therapists' abilities to enhance individuals' self-regulatory behaviors and perceived self-efficacy and to decrease feelings of helplessness become skills useful to physicians in designing a comprehensive and effective intervention plan.

Again, then, actualizing a person's cognitive and behavioral competency – his or her flexibility – represents an important tool in a multidisciplinary approach to intervention. As we turn in the next chapter to consider the embeddedness of individuals in more molar (group and intergenerational) processes, we will see more evidence of the roles of the individual in enhancing human development.

8 Individual and group interdependencies

In this chapter I will focus primarily on the social group as a context for the individual and stress that this context both influences and is influenced by the individual. My goal is to suggest that this bidirectional relation between the individual and the social context within which the individual is embedded may be a key instance of the plasticity of human processes.

Of course, it is possible to focus initially on the group, and not first on the individual; within this more macroscopic emphasis, one may discuss the group as a system of interacting individuals all of whom possess plastic processes and flexibility in influencing and being influenced by one another. In fact, I have discussed elsewhere the nature of, and relation between, these individual and group foci (R. Lerner, 1979, in press) and it is of use to present here some of the key features of these earlier discussions.

A model of individual–context relations

To summarize these other presentations, it is useful to consider the diagram presented in Figure 2. Employing T. C. Schneirla's (1957) terms, this figure illustrates what I described in Chapter 1 as a probabilistic–epigenetic conception of development; in the figure I use the term *maturation* (''Mat.'') to represent endogenous organism changes and the term *experience* (''Exp.'') to denote all stimulative influences acting on the organism over the course of its life span. A conception of interaction levels is used in the figure. The organism's individual developmental history of maturation–experience interactions (what I term Level 1 development – a term analogous to Riegel's [1975] inner biological developmental level) provides a basis of differential organism–environment interactions; in turn, differential experiences accruing from the individual developmental history of organism–environment interactions, or Level 2 development (a term analogous to Riegel's individual psychological developmental level), provides a further basis of Level 1 developmental individuality.

As illustrated in the figure, endogenous maturation–experience interactions

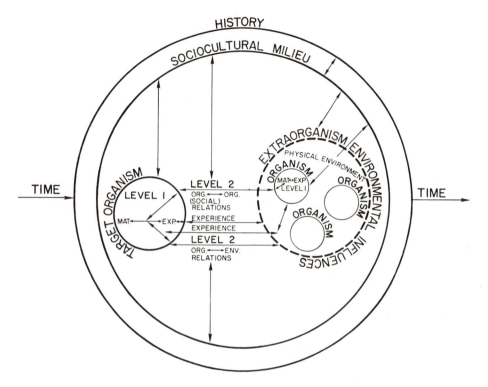

Figure 2. A dynamic interactional model of development. Mat., maturation; Exp; experience; Org., organism; Env., environment. (From Lerner, 1979, p. 277.)

are not discontinuous with exogenous organism–environment interactions. As a consequence of the timing of the interactions among the specific variables involved in an organism's maturation–experience interactions, a basis is provided for an organism's individual distinctiveness. This organism concomitantly interacts differently with its environment as a consequence of this individuality. In turn, these new interactions comprise a component of the organism's further experience and thus serve to further promote its individuality. Endogenous maturation–experience relations provide a basis for organism individuality, and as a consequence differential organism–environment (exogenous) relations develop.

In sum then, the target organism in the figure is unique because of the quality and timing of endogenous, Level 1 maturation–experience interactions; but the experiences that provide a basis of Level 1 development are not discontinuous with other, extraorganism experiences influencing the target individual. The target interacts with environmental influences composed of other organisms (themselves having intraindividual, Level 1 developmental distinctiveness) and of physical variables, which also show individual change over time. Indeed, all tiers of Level 2 – the extraorganism (social), the physical environmental, the sociocultural, and the historical – change over time. Not only does the timing of interactions among variables within and across all tiers provide a distinct experiential context impacting on the developing organism, but this distinctiveness is itself shaped by the individually different organism. In short, in this model I attempt to illustrate the character of probabilistic-epigenetic development.

Some implications of the model

As a consequence of the reciprocity between changes at Levels 1 and 2, two sets of implications arise. The first set of implications emphasizes individual development. Level 2 interchanges will show interindividual differences because of Level 1, intraindividual distinctiveness, and the feedback received as a consequence of these differential interactions will be different among individuals and will promote further Level 1 and Level 2 individuality. This process provides the basis of a circular function (Schneirla, 1957) between an individual and its environment, a function that allows the organism to be an active agent in its own development and allows one to characterize the processes involved in the individual's developmental trajectory as potentially plastic in character.

A second set of implications emphasizes social change. From the model presented in Figure 2 it is clear that there is a systematic connection between individual development and social changes; this connection – already implied in the immediately preceding discussion – becomes evident if one recognizes that (a) the set of individually different and (b) differentially developing organisms living at any one point in time constitute, in effect, the social context and, in part, social change, respectively. In other words (1) if each organism may be characterized at any one point in time as possessing both Level 1 and Level 2 individuality; (2) if these characteristics of individuality change systematically as a consequence of each organism being embedded reciprocally in a context with other individually different organisms; and (3) if the set of all organisms surrounding a given target organism represent the elements of that organism's social world; then (4) this set defines the social context and the changes in this set constitute social change.

This analysis gives both the social context and social change two important features. First, it gives them both an inherent developmental quality; this arises as a consequence of the social context being comprised of developing organisms. Second, this analysis again underscores the contributions of the individual organism, in that the organism, first, affects other organisms (i.e., the social context), and hence elicits feedback to itself, and second, is – in respect to any other target organism – a key element of the social context.

Finally, this analysis provides a rationale for integrating the study of contextual variables marked by concepts such as cohort effects, normative, history-graded influences, and nonnormative events into a comprehensive view of developmental processes. The concepts of "cohort effects," "history-graded influences," and so on are similar in that they are concerned with effects on development other than those typical of contributions made by individual organisms; they are part of the "extraorganism environmental influences" (including the "physical environment") depicted in Figure 2. They denote contextual events that provide commonality across organisms, that shape the experiences of groups of individuals living at particular historical moments. In terms of the present conceptualization, the contextual experiences denoted by these terms comprise an important component of Level 2 stimulative influences: They are components of Level 2 interaction that serve to make organisms living in a context at a given point of time systematically alike. As such, these components of Level 2 are part of the systematic influences on both individual development and on shaping the social context within which organisms transact.

Conclusions. From the perspective of the above model plasticity both contributes to and results from embeddedness in the context. Reciprocal interactions between the individual and context involve functions of the active individual – for example, of his or her cognitions (sense of self or perceived self-efficacy, for instance) and repertoire of specific behaviors and skills – influencing the very context that influences him or her. Recognition of this linkage between the active individual and his or her context opens up numerous avenues of research and intervention, including those attempting to enhance, or alter the impact of, individuals themselves, their inner biological functioning, their context, or linkages among these levels.

Returning our focus to the group as our unit of analysis, we may consider ways in which plasticity characterizing individual developmental processes is also present in more molar units. The links between individual and context outlined above suggest that levels of analysis other than the individual–psychological (e.g., the social context) may undergo developmental change. Making this suggestion more useful is the generic usefulness of a developmental concept, discussed in Chapter 1, that has several features central to a probabilistic-epigenetic perspective: the orthogenetic principle.

As discussed in Chapter 1, Werner (1957; see too Kaplan, 1983) emphasized that orthogenesis is a general, postulative principle of development; according to this principle, whenever development occurs it proceeds from a state of globality, or lack of differentiation, to a state of differentiation, integration, and hierarchic organization. In other words, according to Werner and Kaplan (Kaplan, 1983; Werner, 1948, 1957; Werner and Kaplan, 1956), only changes that follow the pattern described by the orthogenetic principle are to be considered developmental changes. Thus, it is not the level of analysis that is crucial for determining if development has occurred. Rather, it is the features of the changes that take place that determine this. Thus, any unit or level of analysis may undergo changes that follow an orthogenetic sequence.

Indeed, the orthogenetic principle has been used in analyses of the nature and structure of historical changes in society (Brent, 1978a) as well as in theories attempting to integrate the second law of thermodynamics with biosocial change (Prigogine, 1978, 1980). To illustrate the potential developmental plasticity of units of analysis other than the individual–psychological we may use a more modest example than the one of concern to Prigogine. We may focus on the dyad and discuss the characteristics of dyadic relationship development.

Relationship development

Employing the perspective on development of the orthogenetic principle, we may describe the development of dyadic relationships as involving several parameters. Consideration of these parameters leads to a specification of relationship development as involving a progression from an initial global and unidimensional *basis* of interchange to eventual differentiated, multidimensional, multilevel, and hierarchically organized *bases* of interchange.

Developmental level and rate of development of each member of the relationship. The notion of orthogenesis states that processes of development proceed from states of relative globality to ones of relative differentiation and hierarchic integration. Thus, for any dyad one may assess the level (e.g., stage) of differentiation–hierarchization that exists for each member and, through a repeated-measures design, the rate at which each individual is developing through this level. This evaluation will lead to a specification of one of four types of relationships that may exist for a particular dyad at the time of relationship initiation. As can be seen in Figure 3, when a relationship begins the members of the dyad may be at similar or at different levels, which may or may not be progressing at similar rates; relationships may therefore exist at one of four types of symmetry – box 1 representing a relationship of maximum symmetry, box 4 one of least symmetry, and boxes 2 and 3 relationships of intermediate symmetry. Of course, as any of these relationships develops – along the lines I will presently suggest – its placement into another of these symmetry categories is possible. In fact, it may be that depending on the content area of a particular relationship (e.g., employer–employee, graduate student–mentor, mother–child), particular sequences of symmetry occur over the course of the relationship's development.

For example, in the graduate student–mentor relationship, the relationship

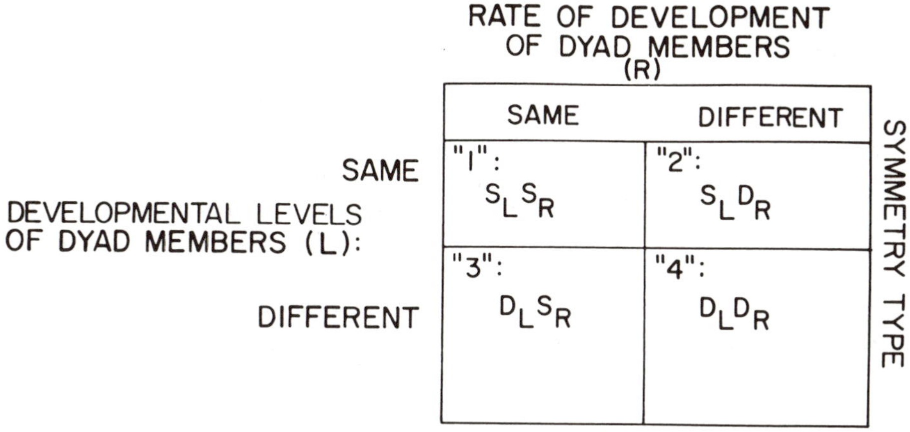

RATE OF DEVELOPMENT
OF DYAD MEMBERS
(R)

	SAME	DIFFERENT	
SAME DEVELOPMENTAL LEVELS OF DYAD MEMBERS (L):	"I": $S_L S_R$	"2": $S_L D_R$	S Y M M E T R Y
DIFFERENT	"3": $D_L S_R$	"4": $D_L D_R$	T Y P E

Figure 3. The type of symmetry at which a relationship exists is dependent on the developmental levels and rates of development of the dyad members. (From Lerner, 1979, p. 286.)

may typically be initiated within symmetry type 4. The student's level of knowledge development is less than that of the mentor (in respect to the domain of graduate study); but while the student is acquiring further knowledge and skills with relative rapidity, as he or she moves (asympototically) toward the level of knowledge of the mentor, the mentor remains at a given level, which is relatively more stable. However, as the relationship progresses it may be locatable in other boxes in Figure 3, and ultimately, if the initial basis of the relationship reaches fruition, it will be locatable in the first box: both student – now former student – and mentor will exist at comparably stable levels of knowledge–skill attainment.

Relationships initiated on the basis of other content reasons may start and proceed through other sequences. Nevertheless, any relationship at any point in its development should be capable of definition in terms of the categories of Figure 3. Although future empirical inquiry will be necessary to indicate where relationships of particular contents begin and where they progress, in terms of their symmetry status over time, and of how deviations from normative symmetry sequencing may affect relationship quality and stability, one may at this point specify two principal parameters of relationship development that should characterize a relationship of any content and of any initial symmetry type. These parameters derive from a further analysis of the orthogenetic nature of development.

Globality to differentiation–hierarchic integration. In the example of the graduate student–mentor relationship it was implied that the basis for relationship initiation was an academic enterprise. The transaction would probably be initiated on the basis of an exchange of knowledge and skills (from the mentor) for capable work and assistance (from the graduate student). However, as the relationship progresses (if it does progress), other reasons for continued transactions may become relevant. The graduate student may want advice about job placement or counseling on how to strike a balance between professional and personal development goals; the mentor may come to regard the graduate student as integral to the further development of his or her work and as a personal friend. Moreover, it should be noted that both initial and new bases for relationship maintenance may exist simultaneously, but that each set of bases may exist at different developmental levels. While the initial dimension of the relationship may still exist at its initial level – or, more probably, a developmentally changed level – any new dimension will upon its emergence follow its own developmental course. One may have considerably differentiated knowledge about someone's intellectual and professional abilities while still having only very general knowledge about his or her personal–intimate characteristics. The point is that new dimensions of a relationship do not automatically and immediately reach the highest developmental level involved in the relationship. A relationship – indeed, a "unit" at even a more molar level of analysis than that of the small group – is best conceived of in multidimensional terms; and each of these components may have its own developmental course. At any one time, then, the dimensions comprising the "unit" of analysis may differ in their developmental levels and rates.

Thus, when a relationship is initiated there is typically a single, general basis for interaction (physical attraction between dyad members, being assigned as a graduate assistant to a professor, giving birth to a child), and relationships exist as relatively global, unidimensional structures at their initiation. But as relationships progress, not only does this general basis become more particularized, but also other dimensions of the relationship emerge as well. A relationship may begin because the dyad members are physically attracted to each other. This attraction may wax, wane, or become more particularized (e.g., "I like her eyes, but not her teeth," "He has a nice body except for his thighs"). And it may become embedded in other, perhaps more salient domains of interchange (e.g., the person is reliable, or disloyal, or affectionate, or aloof).

In addition to such differentiation, other bases for relationship maintenance emerge as a consequence of repeated interchange, and thus relationships develop into multidimensional phenomena. As these other dimensions of interchange become operational, they too follow an orthogenetic course, and thus the multiple dimensions of a developing relationship exist at multiple developmental levels. While each basis of the relationship thus has its own developmental course, all dimensions exist in a hierarchical integration, both within and between dimensions, and they all subserve the functioning of the relationship. In essence, relationships develop toward differentiated, multidimensional, hierarchically integrated levels. Such a developmental progression is illustrated in Figure 4.

In Figure 4 the relationship is initiated at time 1 on the basis of physical attraction between the individuals. At time 2 this attraction has become more differentiated, as attraction to particular body parts comes into play; these less global components may be conceptualized as bipolar dimensions, and thus a particular body part may have a negative weighting. By time 3 this negative–positive differentiation becomes further particularized, and within-dimension hierarchical organization appears; in addition, an aversion domain emerges. By time 4, attraction is high or low to particular body parts, but this attraction domain becomes contrasted with the independent, and now differentiated and hierarchically organized, aversion domain; moreover, both domains have been subordinated to a more general physical dimension. In addition, a social dimension of interchange has emerged, in an orthogenetically initial global state. Development at time 5 involves a further orthogenetic progession of the physical dimension and further differentiation of the social dimension; and at time 6 development involves not only further progression within each of these domains, but also their integration within a superordinate public dimension and the emergence of a personal dimension. Of course, an infinite number of times of relationship development could be depicted, and this means that such development is an open, potentially continually changing system. Moreover, the intervals between depicted times need not be equivalent, and the duration of the relationship is unimportant to the depicted nature of structural progression; that is, both short- and long-term relationships follow an orthogenetic course. Finally, relationships do not have infinite durations, and orthogenetically derived notions will allow us to speak, in a moment, about relationship dissolution.

Such consideration requires analysis of the developmental levels of the dyad members and the type of symmetry implied by these levels. Although a type 4 symmetry (see Figure 3) may characterize numerous relationships, one may conceptualize any symmetry type itself as bipolar and consider the import of the degree of a given type (different developmental level–different rate, for instance) in characterizing a particular relationship.

To understand this point we must first recognize that not only will each dyad member's developmental level and rate of development determine the symmetry type of the relationship, but it will also determine the nature of the orthogenetic progression illustrated in Figure 4. For instance how global each members' conceptual basis for relationship initiation is will determine the level of globality of the initial relationship, the rate of differentiated developmental progressions, and the timing (and nature) of the emergence of other dimensions of the relationship. New mothers will have a more global conception of motherhood than

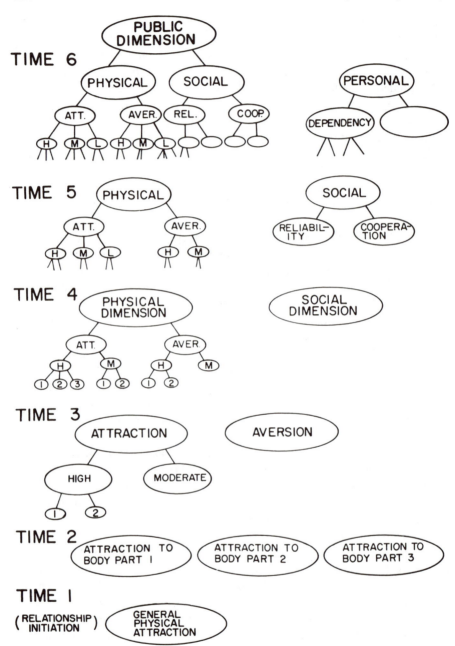

Figure 4. The orthogenetic nature of relationship development. (From Lerner, 1979, p. 289.)

will experienced mothers, and a first romantic relationship is perhaps based on more global and more socially stereotypic conceptions of love and erotic involvement than is a romantic relationship initiated after considerable experience in earlier ones. Either of these relationships (i.e., those involving experienced mothers or experienced lovers) will still begin as relatively global: The particularities of the other dyad member are not yet known, and until they are the new person is necessarily in a relatively general category (e.g., ''my new baby'' or ''my new lover''). However the rate of orthogenetic progression to more advanced levels will be different (e.g., more rapid) for dyads involving these developmentally advanced members. Yet since dyads having developmentally advanced or unadvanced members may be categorized in the same symmetry box when the relationship is initiated, the developmental status of each member of the dyad must be known in order to fully account for all types of variation in a relationship's development (e.g., its rate of differentiation–hierarchization, and hence its rate of sequencing through the four symmetry categories).

More generally, this means that a multilevel perspective must be adopted in order to understand development at any target level of analysis. Here my example was of the need to assess the individual psychological level in order to adequately understand the group. However, it may be necessary to assess small groups in order to understand the community, and similarly, we may have to study communities in order to adequately understand a society. However, lest this point be construed to be an appeal to take a reductionistic, infinite regression route for explanation, let me here note that in addition to assessing the ''lower'' (more molecular) levels comprising any target level, when attempting to understand the target level, one must at the same time assess the more molar levels surrounding the target level. For example, in a later section of this chapter I will review evidence indicating that the social support network surrounding a parent–child dyad may influence the quality of the dyadic relationship (Parke & Tinsley, 1981, 1982). Thus, the point here is that in order to understand the development of any level of analysis, all levels comprising the human condition must be appraised. The full ''ecology of human development'' must be considered (Bronfenbrenner, 1977, 1979).

Oscillation (variability) levels of relationships. A second parameter of relationship development, derivable from our orthogenetic position, may be specified. Not only do the components of relationships become multidimensional, and thus multilevel in developmental status and multirate in progression, but they also become *multidirectional*. The components of relationships cannot be both static and at the same time responsive to the continually changing contingencies in a continually changing environment. If a developmental phenomenon (an organism or a relationship) did not show some flexibility, it would not be aptive (i.e., aiding in survival; Gould & Vrba, 1982; also see Chapter 6) and viable. In fact, it may be the case that one basis of both organism demise (or severe maladaptiveness) and relationship dissolution is that the dimensions (components) of the phenomenon do not exist with degrees of flexibility sufficient to adjust to the changes of the environment. Thus, akin to a notion of dedifferentiation, the dimensions of a relationship may be conceptualized to exist as flexible phenomena, variable in the direction of either more or less globality or differentiation–integration. The level of affection exchanged in a relationship, for example, does not always remain the same, either throughout the relationship's duration or within a particular segment of the relationship. Partners may move from an exchange of love to an exchange of hostility relatively rapidly, or affection may decrease or increase in intensity over a long time span. The point is that oscillation – the variability in behavior associated with a relationship – may be considered for any content domain both within and between temporal segments.

Not only may relationship oscillation occur within a particular content dimension (as in the ups and downs of marital affection), but it also can be seen between content dimensions. Dimensions may differ in their level of globality–differentiation/integration; one may expect, therefore, interdimensional differences in levels of intradimensional variability. For example, it may be hypothesized that the more global the status of a particular dimension (i.e., the more stereotyped the behavior; R. Lerner, 1976), the less the level of oscillation, and that oscillation increases as differentiation proceeds.

One implication of this oscillation parameter is that the components of relationships depicted in Figure 4 should be drawn as theoretical probability distributions rather than as closed loops. An empirical question arises about the appropriate depiction of these distributions. It is logically clear that they need not appear normal, and in fact one might predict that in successful, aptive relationships – for example, marriages having high levels of marital satisfaction (Spanier, 1976) – such distributions would be negatively skewed. For instance, in a highly valued marriage one might expect the preponderant majority of variation in the affection dimension to exist between average and high. Similar predictions could be made for other dimensions of the relationship (e.g., trust, sharing), and one could in fact validate measures of marital satisfaction through interrelation with the various intradimensional oscillation distributions that may exist. Thus, those distributions that approached normality would be associated with marriages having intermediate levels of marital satisfaction; those distributions that were positively skewed would be found in marriages having low satisfaction. Moreover, in any distribution, whatever its form, where variability is minimal, the probability of the relationship's dissolution should be high. Minimally oscillating relationships would not have a sufficient repertoire of responses to employ in the face of the changing demands placed on the rela-

tionship by a changing world (see Riegel, 1976). Alternatively, however, relationships involving maximal oscillation also should be associated with high
probabilities of dissolution; here, continual readjustments and reappraisals would
be involved, and this might mean that the relationship's repertoire of responsiveness would have no more than a random chance of matching the changing
demands placed on it. Accordingly, since either minimal or maximal oscillation
may lead to relationship dissolution, it may be that there exists an oscillation
range that is aptive for relationships of specific developmental characteristics
and attribute domains. In other words, neither the complete absence of flexibility
nor the complete presence of it would seem to be maximally aptive.

A relationship might survive one or even a few minimally or maximally
oscillating dimensions – especially at early levels of relationship development,
when fewer dimensions exist and when they are relatively more global (i.e.,
behaviorally stereotyped) and hence less variable; but no relationship could be
expected to survive when most dimensions, especially key ones, exhibit relatively
minimal or maximal variability. If this should happen, the relationship would
dissolve and, in a sense, return to a state analogous to its initial one. It will exist
in a global state of no-longer-existing. In a sense, all relationships develop toward
this end, as when the death of a dyad member occurs. However, predeath
dissolutions (e.g., divorces) obviously occur. It is the role of future research to
delineate the variables influencing the oscillation characteristics of relationships,
those features making them relatively aptive and successful or unviable and
dissolvable. Some early suggestions were made in this regard by Homans (1974)
and Thibaut and Kelley (1961) when they discussed the roles that such processes
as satiation and alternative sources of reward may play in determining the value
of a particular relationship at a particular point in time.

Conclusions

Not only do individuals follow probabilistic-epigenetic developmental progressions – that is, those involving dynamic interactional change (R. Lerner, 1978,
1979, J. Lerner, 1983) – but the fact that such development is necessarily social
and exchanges are often repeated with the same organisms over time provides
a basis for relationship development also to follow such a course. Moreover, as
with individual ontogeny, relationship development proceeds from a state of
globality, typically initiated on the basis of a single, general dimension of interchange, to a state of increasing differentiation and hierarchic integration.
Numerous dimensions of such open-ended relationships emerge, each following
its own orthogenetic course, and these multiple bases exhibit oscillation characteristics that not only covary with the developmental level of the dimensions

within which they are embedded, but also have import for the relationship's aptive maintenance or dissolution.

Finally, one implication of the individual–context relationship model presented here is that plasticity serves aptive functions not only for the individual, but also for the group and, indeed, for all levels of the social context. In other words, plasticity at the level of the individual may play some role in the aptation of the human group(s) that compose the context in which the individual is embedded. However, as with plasticity at the individual psychological level of anlysis, there may be instances wherein plasticity impedes rather than facilitates aptative functioning (Parke & Tinsley, 1982). We next consider literature from several disciplines that provides some support for and helps clarify this reasoning.

Intergenerational links between the individual and the social group

In their ecologically prototypic milieu individual humans exist in groups (Tobach & Schneirla, 1968). The groups may be composed of individuals from the same generation (e.g., peers), from different generations (e.g., parents and children), and/or may involve social networks not organized on the basis of age (e.g., community or professional groups). In this section, the aptational significance of plasticity for both the individual and the group will be illustrated by focusing on features of intergenerational relations. To begin this discussion it is useful to make several points about the nature of the individual, his or her social context, and the development of their interrelations:

1. As discussed in Chapter 6, processes linking the person to the group have been selected in evolution (Fisher, 1982a; Gould, 1977; Lovejoy, 1981). But given a dynamically interactive, probabilistic-epigenetic view of biology–context relations (summarized in part in Chapters 1 and 2 and preceding sections of this chapter), these processes do not exist fully developed, preformed, or innate in the newborn (see also Gottlieb, 1970, 1976a, b; R. Lerner, 1978, 1979). Accordingly, those interested in human development must understand how the processes that link the individual to its context change across ontogeny. At the individual psychological level of analysis, reinforcement processes, cognitive developmental processes, and social relational processes, such as attachment and dependency, may *all* be involved.

2. Because of the link between individual aptation and social functioning, the group is necessary for the individual's survival. For example, Hogan, Johnson and Emler (1978) point out that "social living is the key to man's evolutionary success" (p. 3), and in regard to behavioral functioning (to them largely *moral* functioning) they note that if the societal "rules are ignored, social living is impossible. If a person seriously does not care about the survival of his or her

culture, then that person would not be immoral in an absolute sense – but that person would be either criminal or insane'' (p. 3). Thus, in this view, personal survival depends on supporting, at least in part, the social context within which one is embedded.

3. A third point, however, leads us to focus on the plasticity of an individual's processes. Just as the individual needs the group, the group needs the individual, and a singular individual at that. The individual is necessary for the group's survival (e.g., to populate it and perpetuate the techniques it has used for survival). That is, as Brim and Kagan (1980, p. 19) have put the issue, ''Society must transform the raw material of individual biology into persons suitable for the activities and requirements of society'' (see also Ryder, 1965). For example, Hogan et al. (1978) point out that, ''the process of transmitting culture across human generations is fundamental to human survival'' (p. 6), although ''the rules are important not in themselves but because they serve to legitimize, sanction, and promote certain behaviors that are essential to the operation and survival of culture'' (p. 4). Thus, the ''tendencies toward ritualization, codification, and organization make social living predictable and more efficient'' (p. 6). Simply, these rules enhance the aptiveness of social functioning. Similarly, Baumrind (1978, p. 66) has suggested that ''the function of social rules, whether conventional or moral, is to coordinate the individual's immediate prudential or hedonistic aims with (1) his or her longer-range interests; and (2) the interests, shorter- and longer-range, of his or her primary group and impersonal collective.'' Accordingly, she notes that social–moral sanctions

are simply metaconventions that the human species has evolved in adapting to and mastering its environment. When conditions of long-range survival change, then moral sanctions change with them. Moral principles and their development, like other social rules and their development, arise from concrete cultural-historical conditions. (P. 69)

Similarly, Hogan et al. (1978, pp. 6–7) note that a major evolutionary component of the sociocultural context is

a set of child-rearing practices that serves to transmit whatever technological wisdom the group has evolved, together with the values necessary to apply that wisdom effectively. Thus we have a feedback loop consisting of environmental demands, the cultural resources developed in response to these demands, and child-rearing practices which provide for cultural transmission and development of the character type best suited to the environmental demands.

But there is another, essential feature to the link between individuals and their social context. As noted by both Hogan et al. and Baumrind, it is clear that the context changes. If the rules of a social group represent a specification of the content of exchanges that people and their institutions must make with their context in order for adaptation to occur (i.e., maintenance and perpetuation, or reproduction), then both person and group must ''institutionalize'' flexibility as well as stability. Hogan et al. (1978, p. 3) make this point when they note that "the moral rules that make social living possible only tell us what kinds of behavior were necessary for survival in the past; they may not be valid for the future. Moreover, the conditions under which any social group lives may change. Thus cultures must always be open to the possibilities for change and innovation."

Thus, the integration of flexible individuals into the social group enhances the group's flexibility and hence its ability to adapt to changes in the forces impinging on it. This link between individual and group flexibility is made possible by the plasticity of individual–social context relations; however, if the social context supporting both individual and group is to be perpetuated and not only maintained, this link must be institutionalized (and to this extent constrained, in that institutions may not be as readily flexible as the individuals living within the institution). Such institutionalization must involve intergenerational transmission across the flow of succeeding cohorts if adaptive progressions are to occur. Information from both evolutionary biology and from life course sociology allows us to appreciate what may be involved.

Parent–child relations and human neoteny

Sociologists and various human developmentalists point out that plasticity is needed on both macro and micro levels of analysis (e.g., Bengtson & Troll, 1978; Haan, 1981; Riley, 1979a, b). Haan (1981) notes that although individuals may be inextricably linked to the group, they strive to see themselves as individuals, and John Clausen (cited in Brim & Kagan, 1980, p. 17) observes that "the natural state of the person is to be in the process of becoming something different while in many respects remaining the same" (e.g., like him- or herself in earlier developmental periods and like others in his or her group). Sociologically such an orientation – one counter to complete social molding (Hartup, 1978) – must occur if individuals and their society are to be maximally aptive. An individual member of a new birth cohort enters a social system composed of already existing cohorts. If all a person could or would do is replicate the behaviors that were aptive for that older cohort, then, given a changed context, that person would not be aptive (see Riley, 1978). A society composed of such people would not survive. Thus, the social context has an investment in an individual. Society needs members of the new cohort to maintain and perpetuate it. Accordingly, it is necessary to promote, foster, and tolerate variation from the existing context's behavioral repertoire.

Gould's (1977) ideas from evolutionary biology about human neoteny provide a basis for understanding the biological and aptive bases of these relations among members of succeeding age cohorts. Neoteny provides aptive advantages for members of both older and younger generations. Considering children first, the neoteny of the human results in human newborns being perhaps the most dependent organisms found among placental mammalian infants (Gould, 1977). Moreover, their neoteny means that this dependency is extraordinarly prolonged, and this requires intense parental care of the child for several years. The plasticity of childhood processes, which persists among humans for more than a decade, thus entails a history of necessarily close contact with adults and places an "adaptive premium ... on learning (as opposed to innate response) ... unmatched among organisms" (Gould, 1977, p. 401). Gould agrees with de Beer (1959, p. 930) that for the human, "delay in development enabled him to develop a larger and more complex brain, and the prolongation of childhood under conditions of parental care and instruction consequent upon memory-stored and speech-communicated experience, allowed him to benefit from *a more efficient apprenticeship for his conditions of life*" (italics added). In other words, the neoteny of humans, their prolonged childhood dependency on others, and their embeddedness in a social context composed of members of the older generation who both protect them and afford them the opportunity to actualize their potential plasticity allow members of a new birth cohort to adapt to the conditions and influences particular to their historical epoch.

Of course, such development in a new cohort has evolutionary significance for members of the older cohort as well. Gould (1977) points out that neoteny and the protracted period of dependent childhood may have led to the evolution of features of adult human (parental) behavior. The presence of young and dependent children and the need to effectively support and guide them require adults to be organized in their adult–adult and adult–child interactions. Furthermore, since the period of childhood dependency is so long, it is likely that human history tended to involve the appearance of later-born children before earlier-born ones achieved full independence (Gould, 1977). Gould (1977, p. 403) sees such a tendency as facilitating the emergence of pair bonding and identifies "in delayed development a primary impetus for the origin of the human family."

Parent–child relations and intergenerational "stakes"

Neoteny and prolonged childhood development may be important to adults for another reason. Having an extended period of time to socialize their children, parents may therefore be afforded a period within which to insure that their children will grow up to want to protect, maintain, and perpetuate the society and social order in which the parents invested – in which, in other words, they have what Bengtson and his colleagues (Bengtson & Kuypers, 1971; Bengtson & Troll, 1978) term a "generational stake." That is, not only will children perpetuate parental genes, but they may also be generally regarded by parents as cherished "investments" in those customs, mores, and ideals that the parents hold dear to themselves, including having a family and rearing children. Thus, it is of aptive significance for children to actualize their potential for plasticity (so that they achieve compatibility with their particular historical influences); and it is in the parents' interest, as members of the older generation, to facilitiate this plastic development so that society as a whole will be more aptive with differentially plastic individuals present.

However, the parents, as members of the older cohort, will not "permit" too much variability from their orientation, or else their "generational stake" would be diminished significantly. Nevertheless, the new cohort will rarely if ever completely overthrow the inculcation orientation of the older cohort, because:

1. They have their own "generational stake" in the older cohort – they may need them for the production of certain goods or for the presence of certain skills they themselves do not have;
2. There is much in the older cohort's repertoire that still remains functional, that is, that shows cross-cohort adaptive significance;
3. There is meaning (e.g., valuation) placed on these older others; and
4. There are empathic, attachment, or dependency processes that may be engaged in intergenerational relations.

In sum, avoiding complete social molding, individuals maintain their individual flexibility, which enhances their aptiveness and that of their social context. Thus, there is a "dialectic" between individual (I) and group (G) processes:

1. I's goals $=$ G's goals (because of the social nature of individual behavior); but
2. I's goals $\neq$ (differ from) G's goals (for example, because I wants to see self as an individual; Haan, 1981); but
3. Because in supporting I's individuality, or potential for individuality (i.e., plasticity), G's goals – of maintenance *and* of perpetuation – will be served (i.e., there will be a population of Is who are flexible enough to meet potentially new contextual demands), it is again the case that
4. I's goals $=$ G's goals.

Individuals and the organismic collective

As implied earlier in this chapter, individuals do not typically exist as members of only one group. Individuals are responsive to and belong to multiple groups. Simply put, the social context is not unidimensional. That is, although the social context is integrated (e.g., interdependent), it is also differentiated. Thus, in a sense, each individual may be unique by virtue of his or her being a "composite" of those reciprocal relations maintained toward an array of segments of the social context. Individuals' views of themselves as unique may, in this way, be quite veridical. They will therefore make a distinct or variable contribution to the society and in this way enhance the overall context's level of flexibility.

Brent (1978a, p. 23) has made a compatible point:

A dialectical relationship exists between the tendency toward specialization of each individual member of an organismic collective during the course of individual development (e.g., ontogenesis) and the tendency toward adaptation of the organismic collective-as-a-whole to a shifting set of environmental opportunities and constraints during the course of its development (e.g., phylogenesis). The general principle is this: As each individual within an organismic collective becomes increasingly more specialized in the unique niche which he/she occupies in the collective, the collective-as-a-whole becomes increasingly more flexible in its ability to adapt to its changing environment. Put in other terms: *The specialization of individuals within an organismic collective is the concrete realization at the micro-structural level of differentiation of the organismic collective-as-a-whole at the macrostructural level.*

Moreover, Brent points out that social context maintenance and perpetuation depend on intergenerational relations that involve the continuation of past aptation strategies along with the promotion of plasticity, especially in the newer cohorts. He argues that

each organismic collective in order to survive and prosper must fulfill three kinds of functions simultaneously. First, it must maximize the efficiency with which it fulfills those functions essential to its maintenance and survival as an entity under some existing set of environmental conditions. Second, it must maximize the facility with which it can maintain its own stability in the face of changes in these environmental conditions. And, third, it must at the same time maintain the ability to expand into new environmental niches as the opportunity for such expansions arise. (Pp. 24–25)

Brent indicates that the biocultural ''solution'' to this problem involves a situation wherein

each phylogenetically younger structural cohort embeds all of the older cohorts in a layer of protective environment which allows the older to continue to function in a stable and 'traditional' manner while permitting the organism, i.e., collective-as-a-whole, to expand into new environmental niches in which the older cohorts, by themselves, could never survive or function. (Pp. 27–28)

Conclusions. A focus on intergenerational relations indicates the aptive role of flexibility at both individual and group levels of analysis, flexibility that is an outcome of the plastic processes linking individuals to their social context. Moreover, while members of different generations have many converging developmental interests, certain features of their respective functioning are distinctive – and necessarily so, given that each generation experiences somewhat different aptational influences. For example, children and adolescents may seek to enhance their flexibility and individual singularity; in large part, the reciprocal socialization interactions between them and their parents may be used to develop their unique self-conceptions, identities, ideology, skills, and behaviors. In turn, parents may be seeking in large part to inculcate in their children those attitudes, values, and behavioral orientations in which they themselves have invested. Problems between children and adolescents and their parents may be complicated by a failure to understand and discriminate between forces that bring children and adults together and ontogenetic-period-specific ones that may separate them. Educators, family counselors, and family sociologists may find it useful to make such discriminations, however, in assessing the nature of the issues that confront them in their attempts to enhance individual and/or family functioning.

For instance, as the child develops toward increasing independence, it may become increasingly more difficult to insure compliance with necessary, adult-imposed regimens. Cases in point are the difficulty physicians may encounter in insuring that seizure-prone adolescents take necessary medication at prescribed times and the problems that counselors of sexually active, unmarried young adolescents may have in insuring that birth control is regularly and correctly used. Knowledge of the character of individual and group interdependencies and of the aptive significance of intergenerational relations should facilitate the development of plans for preventive as well as remedial interventions. For instance, building on the flexibility of both parents and their children (provided by neotenous human evolution), anticipatory socialization interventions may be instituted.

Finally, however, we should note that the intergenerational perspective we have been taking in this section is not the only one useful for understanding how individual and group interdependencies may provide a basis of plasticity in human functioning. Members of other generations represent only one component of the social network that may surround an individual. Therefore, we may draw also from information in the social networks literature (e.g., Bronfenbrenner, 1977, 1979; Parke, 1977, 1978, 1979, 1981a, 1981b; Parke, Hymel, Power, & Tinsley, 1980; Parke & Tinsley, 1981, 1982) to gain insight into other bases. Moreover, this altered focus will allow us to emphasize once again the "double-edged sword" nature of human plasticity: we will see that the embeddedness of individuals in their social network involves plastic interpersonal processes, but that such processes may be associated with either positive or negative outcomes for the individual.

The individual in his or her social network

Parke and Tinsley (1982) review an increasing number of models relating individuals to their social network that involve a "recognition of the reciprocity of families as socializing agents embedded in social networks, both directly and indirectly influencing and being influenced by interactions within and outside the family" (p. 1).

For example, in respect to the mother–infant dyad, Parke and Tinsley note that among the models currently guiding research and intervention are those that view this dyad as embedded in social systems such as the mother–father–child family system (e.g., Belsky, 1981; Parke, Power, & Gottman, 1979; Pedersen,

1981), formal and informal support systems (e.g., Bronfenbrenner, 1979; Cochran & Brassard, 1979; Parke, 1977), and the cultural system (LeVine, 1977; Parke, Grossman, & Tinsley, 1981).

Among the many models currently guiding research in this area are those that focus on the father's influence on the mother–infant dyad (Lamb, 1981); such models stress that there are three dyadic interactions in a three-person family (mother–child, father–child, and mother–father) and one triadic one, and that one must attend to the relationships among these different family subsystems. In this regard, Pedersen (1981, pp. 313–14) notes that

father influences appear vastly more complex when viewed in a perspective of a family system. Viewing the mother–infant and father–infant relationship in a psychological vacuum is a fiction of convenience that may have been serviceable in guiding past research, but it will have to be replaced by more ambitious attempts to conceptualize a broader range of experiences and more complex notions of psychological causation within the family.

In turn, Parke and Tinsley (1981) note that systems outside the family influence functioning within it; for example, social support systems that aid the father in his parent role enable him to facilitate the mother's parent role.

Parke and Tinsley (1982) note that from the features of such models one may infer that the ability of an individual or a group (e.g., a family) to adjust to a stressful event is in part mediated by the "unit's" position within such levels of social organization and by access to and use of the various social supports found therein. A study by Crockenberg (1981) supports the view of Parke and Tinsley and also presages a discussion (of temperament) in the next chapter. Crockenberg (1981) studied the influence of infant irritability, maternal responsiveness, and maternal social support on the development of secure and anxious infant–mother attachments at one year of age. Social support was found to be the best predictor of secure attachment, and social support was most important for mothers with irritable infants. In fact, although evidence was found linking maternal unresponsiveness with the development of anxious attachment, Crockenberg also found that social support mitigated these effects by providing the infant with a responsive substitute. Summarizing these results, Crockenberg (1981) observes:

support had its strongest effect on the irritable babies and their mothers, [suggesting] that the availability of social support is particularly critical when the family is under particular stress ... children who are irritable or in other ways less rewarding/more demanding of their parents are at risk for later developmental difficulty only if their environments are deficient in meeting their special needs. (pp. 862, 864)

Accordingly, Crockenberg (1981) indicates that social support may enhance aptive developmental functioning and help the individual avoid "at risk" status if the support matches – or (as will be discussed in Chapter 9) provides a "goodness of fit" with – the individual's personal characteristics (which in the Crockenberg, 1981, study, as well as in many of the studies to be discussed in Chapter 9, involve a temperament dimension – irritability in this case). However, the converse of the above implication of Crockenberg's view should be noted also, and so we consider it next.

The social network: facilitative versus impeding influences

One may interpret the results of Crockenberg's (1981) study as indicating that if there is not a good fit between social support and the individual's attributes, then embeddedness in a particular social system can hamper the person's aptive development. Parke and Tinsley (1982) make this point explicitly: "It should be noted that community influence, regardless of its form, can be either positive or negative; this view stands in contrast to the view that high degree of connectedness with community resources is, *ipso facto*, necessarily positive (p. 10).

A report by Wahler (1980) presents data that support the view of Parke and Tinsley. Mothers in 31 families with problematic parent–child relations were given training in behavior modification techniques with the goal of giving them the skills to act as sources of reinforcement in the potential resolution of these problems (Wahler, 1980). Training (treatment) success or failure was associated with the type of social network within which the mother was embedded. As described by Wahler (1980, p. 191), "the treatment failure group had fewer community interactions and these few were predominantly with kinfolk and helping-agency representatives. In contrast, the more socially gregarious treatment-success mothers spent the bulk of their extrafamily time with friends."

In sum, Wahler's findings illustrate that the success or failure of an intervention targeted at our individual is dependent on the nature of the individual's social context. Thus, Crockenberg's (1981) research gives us a basis for the inference that developmental processes of the individual – even those that may enhance flexibility of functioning – may not be aptive unless they provide a fit with the features of the social system within which the person exists. And from Wahler's report we see that the social context may allow or constrain the success of an intervention that is designed to increase flexible, aptive functioning.

Taken together then, the presentation of Parke and Tinsley (1982) and the data reported by Crockenberg and Wahler underscore the "double-edged sword" character of plasticity: Not all changes that are associated with greater plasticity need be aptive for the individual; features of the context and the goodness of fit between these contextual conditions and individual characteristics influence how aptive a change may be. Thus, social context links, whether they be between members of different generations or between a person and his or her peer, community, or professional group, may either impede or facilitate change and development; embeddedness in one level can work for or against change produced by agents at other levels.

Conclusions

The challenge for researchers and interventionists is to discover how the links between the individual and the multiple levels of his or her context may impede or facilitate the development of particular aptive and/or valued characteristics. To meet this challenge one needs theoretical models encompassing the multilevel, multivariate links between individuals and their context.

One such model, focusing specifically on child and parent development, is presented in Figure 5 (cf. R. Lerner & J. Lerner, 1984). Here I have tried to illustrate the complex nature of intraindividual, interindividual, social network, and still broader contextual relations. Children and adults – as parents – have evolved to exist in a reciprocal relationship (Gould, 1977; Johanson & Edey, 1981; Lovejoy, 1981). At the same time each of these members of the dyad are not only interacting; they are also both developing. And the development of each is, at least in part, both a product and a producer of the development of the other. Moreover, both parent and child are embedded in a broader social network, and each has reciprocal relations with this network, too. Furthermore, both child and parent are much more than just unirole or undifferentiated organisms. The child may also be a sibling, a peer, and a student; the parent may also be a spouse, a worker, a peer, and an adult child. Both parent and child have temperaments, cognitions, emotions, interests, attitudes, values, demands, physical and health characteristics, and so on. And each of these attributes may be influenced by the intraindividual developmental status of the remaining attributes, as well as by the developmental status of one or all of the other dyad member's attributes.

The bidirectional relations described in Figure 5 may be seen to be identical in general form to those illustrated in Figure 2. In turn, the relations shown in both Figures 2 and 5 may be seen to be akin to those presented earlier in Figure 1 (Chapter 6). Indeed, in my view Figures 2 and 5 are just "translations" of the earlier figure into ones stressing ontogenetic, as opposed to evolutionary, relations.

However, let me emphasize that the model in Figure 5 serves only as a descriptive summary of the evolutionary and ontogenetic person–social context relations that I have discussed in Chapter 6 and in the present chapter. In addition, while I do not believe that it would be useful or even possible to do research

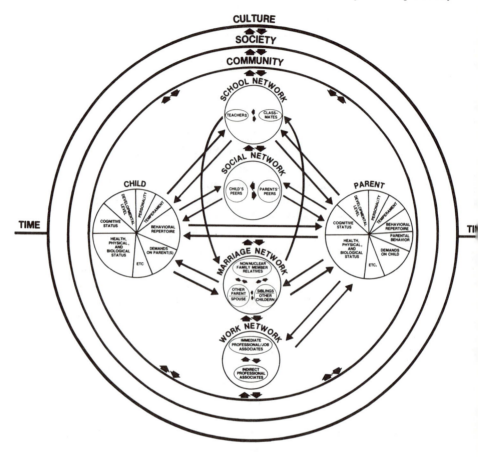

Figure 5. A dynamic interactional model of child and parent development.

testing the model as a whole, my view is that the model constitutes a specification of the domain within which future theory and research about individual–social context relations should be generated. It guides the selection of individual and ecological variables in one's research and provides parameters about the generalizability of one's findings. Finally, the model is prescriptive for theory. It stresses that one should formulate ideas stressing the relation between a particular feature of an individual and a specific aspect of his or her context.

As has been suggested repeatedly in the preceding chapters of this book, the set of concepts associated with the life-span view of human development may be of use in such necessarily multilevel, model-testing research and in intervention as well. In the next chapter of this book I will briefly indicate the use of the life-span perspective in furthering multidisciplinary research and intervention aimed at enhancing human development. As an illustration, I will emphasize research that, like that of Crockenberg (1981), stresses that the fit between individual and context is central for understanding whether an individual's changes will result in his or her aptive functioning.

9   Toward future multidisciplinary efforts

The life-span view of human development emphasizes the potential for change across life. As such, plasticity is a key idea in this perspective. Plasticity is seen to arise because the levels of analysis involved in human life are not only themselves comprised of plastic processes but also because each level is reciprocally interactive with (embedded in) all others. Change at one level promotes changes at the others.

In this book I have reviewed theory and data from levels of analysis ranging from the genetic to the intergenerational, social network, and cultural. Although this review is not exhaustive, I believe that the evidence I discussed allows several conclusions to be made. First, at all levels of analysis, the variables considered are part of other processes, and means to manipulate the nature of these variables, or at least change their impact or outcome, are often available. Physical therapy with cerebral palsy children may not result in motor improvement above a "just noticeable difference." However, the parents of children receiving such therapy may be made more optimistic, may feel less guilty or anxious, and may therefore enter into more positive interactions with their child; the child's feelings about him- or herself may in turn be positively altered, and this change will encourage the continuation of the parents' positive interactions with the child. Although the physical features of the child's functioning may still remain largely unaltered, because the child is embedded in a positive reciprocal relation with his or her context, the intervention may have a quite useful, albeit indirect (and perhaps unintended) effect. Thus, the effect of the motor disability on the child and his or her family would be altered.

Second, the processes to which variables at each level of analysis are related are often ones lying at other levels of analysis; for instance, neuroanatomical changes are linked to (moderated by) the psychosocial stimulus history of the organism, and neurochemical transmission processes are linked to (influence) cognitive functioning and change at various points across life. Third, these links among levels of analysis often involve bidirectional or reciprocal interactions.

To illustrate, recall that in Chapter 5 we considered the role of dietary inter-

146

ventions in altering neurotransmitter levels in the brain and indicated that dietary manipulations affect other features of the organism in addition to the neurochemical balance. Weindruch and Walford (1982) point out that rats given restricted diets from about the age of weaning (3 to 6 weeks) show extended mean and maximum survival times, deceleration in the rate of aging, and a decreased incidence or delayed onset of several diseases of old age – for example, spontaneous cancers and decreased immunologic responsivity. Weindruch and Walford have reported that similar changes can be produced when dietary manipulation of rodents is begun in their middle age, and thus have provided evidence that the organism remains open to substantial physiological enhancement well beyond early life. Specifically, Weindruch and Walford began a dietary restriction program ("undernutrition without malnutrition") among middle-aged (12- to 13-month-old) mice. These mice averaged 10–20% increases in mean and maximum survival times compared to control mice; moreover, the food restriction inhibited spontaneous lymphoma.

Findings such as these, if extended to humans, provide a rationale for a multidisciplinary approach to intervention, one based on reciprocal relations among levels. Behavioral and cognitive–behavioral therapists, for example, could help clients maintain an "undernutrition without malnutrition" dietary regimen, designed by a nutritionist, as part of an intervention program of prevention (e.g., against cancer) or enhancement (e.g., of longevity).

Finally, a fourth point may be made. Because of plasticity there is always a potential for intervention; and because of the reciprocal links among levels of analysis such intervention appropriately may, and perhaps should, be multidisciplinary.

Of course, few scientists are expert enough to plan such work alone. Fewer still are capable of conducting the basic research from which multidisciplinary interventions should derive. Thus, collaborative research and intervention efforts must be initiated. Such work should not be considered either a luxury (something to do after "important" scientific concerns have been addressed) or, as may often be the case, an activity of those interested not in basic issues but in "softer," more humanistic, or only applied concerns.

If we take seriously the life-span conception of plasticity – that is, that it not only enables but also derives from reciprocal interactions among all levels of analysis comprising human life – then multidisciplinary research, of the sort I have suggested throughout this book, *is* research aimed at understanding basic processes. And if the plasticity of humans is the hallmark of the species, what makes us unique, or creates those characteristics that, in combination, comprise the signature of an organism being human, then interventions aimed at enhancing plasticity are of paramount significance.

What may such intervention entail? Throughout this book I have given examples of the sorts of research questions and potential interventions that seem appropriate and useful given the state of knowledge at a particular level of analysis. Here, let me note some general considerations. Before any intervention is initiated, assessment must take place (Kendall, 1981). However, the task of assessment suggested by a life-span orientation is as multidisciplinary as any intervention might be. At the very least, variables from four levels of analysis must be assessed: (1) inner biological (e.g., genetic-, neurotransmitter-, endo-crine-, and nutrient-related) variables; (2) individual psychological (e.g., cog-nitive, affective, and behavioral) variables; (3) sociocultural, including ecological (e.g., family, social network, and societal), as well as physical environmental, variables; and (4) historical variables (e.g., variables relating to intergenerational transmission and social change). Moreover, in view of the fact that variables from all levels of analysis are not static, but rather may be seen as change processes, variables from all levels must be understood as developmental ones. We must assess the status of developmental trajectories, not only because this will give us a more accurate depiction of the variables with which we are dealing, but also because it will broaden our range of potential timings for our interven-tions. We may adopt an ahistorical (i.e., immediate) intervention, one which deals with either proximal or distal targets, and one which is aimed at either remediation or enhancement. In addition, we may adopt a historical (i.e., de-layed) intervention, and therefore one focused on distal targets, and one which is aimed at enhancement *or* prevention.

An example of both the obvious complexity and potential use of life-span–based assessment and intervention may suffice to illustrate the precise sorts of efforts for which I am calling. Consider a child in the middle elementary school grades who, with no apparent mental retardation or physical, medical, or familial problems, is obtaining lower and lower grades in mathematics. The sorts of assessments I have suggested might reveal:

1. Subtle neurotransmitter deficits (an inner biological assessment) impacting on either short-term or long-term memory (individual psychological assessments);
2. Nutritional deficiencies (an inner biological assessment) resulting from either poor eating habits (an individual psychological assessment) or nutritionally insufficient food available to the child as a consequence of family socioeconomic status (a sociocultural assessment) or intergenerationally transmitted dietary customs (a historical assessment);
3. Inappropriate self-statements – for example, inaccurately perceived self-efficacy (an individual psychological assessment), resulting from being the target of peer or familial psychological abuse or neglect (a sociocultural assessment); or
4. Differential socialization, as a consequence of the sex of the child and of sex role stereotypes or as a consequence of peer pressures, teacher behaviors, or school structure (again, sociocultural assessments).

In turn, appropriate interventions for each of these four outcomes of assessment might respectively involve: (1) administration of dietary precursors of the deficient neurotransmitter and/or memory-training regimens; (2) nutritional supplements, behavioral or cognitive–behavioral therapy, counseling about or referral to private or public financial assistance programs, or family therapy; (3) cognitive–behavioral therapy, family counseling, community support services, or court/police referral; or (4) public policy or social change interventions aimed at altering sex-associated differential socialization.

That linkages such as those illustrated in the assessment and intervention aspects of this example are neither improbable nor impossible has, I believe, been evidenced by much of the information I have reviewed. However, in further support of my argument, I will illustrate how a specific topic in human development may be approached using the perspective called for here. Specifically, this illustration draws on points made in Chapter 8's discussion of the embeddedness of individuals in a social network. As indicated in my presentation of the work of Parke and Tinsley (1981, 1982) and of Crockenberg (1981), the social network may enhance aptive developmental functioning, and help the individual avoid "at risk" status if there is a congruence, match, or "good fit" between the features of the social context and the person's characteristics of individuality. There is considerable compatability between this notion of "goodness of fit" and the ideas I have been presenting about multidisciplinary research and intervention. Thus, I will next discuss a model of individual–context "goodness of fit" and illustrate my points by drawing on the substantive literature most pertinent to this model – that is, theory and research about temperamental individuality.

A "goodness-of-fit" model of person–context relations: the sample case of temperament

The conception that the relationships between an organism and its context must involve congruence, match, or simply fit in order for adaptive transactions to exist is an idea traceable at least to Darwin (1859). As explained by White (1968), this idea has permeated American and to some extent European social science, albeit in formulations as seemingly diverse as those of G. S. Hall (1904), Clark Hull (1952), and George Herbert Mead (1934). Several literatures suggest that a goodness-of-fit approach is useful. Among adults, degree of fit between personality characteristics and demands of the work setting predict both physical and mental health (e.g., French, Rodgers, & Cobb, 1974; Harrison, 1978; Kohn & Schooler, 1979). In adolescence, levels of personality fit with pressures of the high school setting covary with school alienation and involvement and with school misbehavior (Kulka, 1979; Kulka, Klingel, & Mann, 1980). Among children, the degree to which one's physical characteristics fit with others' attitudes regarding facial and bodily attractiveness covaries with personal, interpersonal, and academic behavior in the elementary school setting (e.g., Sorrell & Nowak, 1981).

In infancy, data pertinent to the mother–infant dyad, reviewed in the preceding chapter, are consistent with the goodness-of-fit concept. Crockenberg (1981) found that irritable babies – babies that place greater caregiving demands on their mothers – are at risk for later problems only if the babies' environments do not meet their specific needs; that is, these babies were at risk only when there was a poor fit between their specific (temperamental) characteristics and the support resources for these characteristics available in their context.

A version of the goodness-of-fit idea that has been attracting increasing attention in the human development literature is provided by the psychiatrists Thomas and Chess (1977). Their goodness-of-fit model, which may be traced in specific form to Henderson (1913), indicates that aptive developmental outcomes are most likely when a person's physical and behavioral characteristics are consonant with the demands of the physical and social developmental context. However, the degree of goodness of fit present at one point in time may not be present at another time. The person's physical and behavioral attributes may be developing, and the demands of the context may also change. In addition, demands may take many forms; for example, there may be demands placed on a person as a consequence of (1) the attitudes or expectations of others; (2) the behavioral attributes of others; and (3) the physical features of a setting (e.g., the presence or absence of access ramps in the case of a wheelchair-bound person).

Because of this changing complexity, Thomas and Chess's (1977) goodness-of-fit model has been extended beyond its unitemporal, descriptive character (J. Lerner, 1983; J. Lerner & Lerner, 1983). Attention has begun to be paid to the processes by which children may change themselves or be changed to meet the demands of changing and multiple contexts; in turn, there has also been concern with the processes by which children may change contextual demands to fit their attributes (J. Lerner & R. Lerner, 1983). This work builds on the theory and research of Schneirla (1957), specifically in regard to his ideas concerning circular functions and self-stimulation in ontogeny. These ideas were seen to represent the foundation of the probabilistic-epigenetic model of person–social context relations discussed in Chapter 8 (and illustrated in Figure 2). That is, these ideas, which entail an appreciation of the contextual significance of a person's characteristics of individuality, indicate that as a consequence of characteristics of physical individuality (e.g., sex, body type, or facial attractiveness; Berscheid & Walster, 1974) and/or psychological individuality (e.g., in regard to conceptual tempo, or temperament; Kagan, 1966; Thomas & Chess, 1977), people promote differential reactions in their socializing others; these reactions may feed back to people, increase the individuality of their developmental milieu, and provide a basis for their further development.

Through the establishment of such "circular functions" in ontogeny (Schneirla, 1957), people may be conceived of as producers of their own development (R. Lerner & Busch-Rossnagel, 1981). However, this circular functions idea needs to be extended; that is, in and of itself the notion is mute regarding the specific characteristics of the feedback (e.g., its positive or negative valence) that an organism will receive as a consequence of its individuality. However, the nature of the reactions evoked in others and the concomitant feedback received can be understood by again invoking the goodness-of-fit idea. Children whose characteristics (e.g., in terms of physical attractiveness, behavioral style, or temperament) are consonant with contextual pressures (for example, attitudes, values, or expectations of their parents, peers, or teachers) will evoke positive reactions in these others and receive favorable feedback. In other words, just as a person brings his or her characteristics of individuality to a particular social setting, there are demands placed on the person by virtue of the social and physical components of the setting, demands that may take the form of:

1. Attitudes, values, or stereotypes held by others in the context regarding the person's attributes (physical or behavioral characteristics);
2. The attributes (usually behavioral) of others in the context with whom the child must coordinate, or fit, his or her attributes (also, in this case, usually behavioral) for adaptive interactions to exist; or
3. The physical characteristics of a setting (e.g., the presence or absence of access ramps for the wheelchair-bound) that require the person to possess certain attributes (again, usually behavioral abilities) for the most efficient interaction within the setting to occur.

The person's individuality in differentially meeting these demands provides a basis for the feedback he or she gets from the socializing environment. For example, considering the demand "domain" of attitudes, values, or stereotypes, teachers and parents may have relatively individual and distinct expectations about behaviors desired of their students and children, respectively. Teachers may want students who show little distractibility, since they would not want attention diverted from the lesson by the activity of other children in the classroom. Parents, however, might desire their children to be moderately distractible – for example, when they require their children to move from television watching to dinner or to bed. Children whose behavioral individuality was either generally distractible or generally not distractible would thus differentially meet the demands of these two contexts. Problems of adaptation to school or to home might thus develop as a consequence of a child's lack of match (goodness of fit) in either or both settings.

Similarly, considering the second type of contextual demands – those that arise as a consequence of the behavioral characteristics of others in the setting – problems of fit might occur when a child who is highly irregular in his biological functions (e.g., eating, sleep–wake cycles, toileting behaviors) interacts in a family setting composed of highly regular and behaviorally scheduled parents and siblings. In turn, considering the third type of contextual demands – those that arise as a consequence of the physical characteristics of a setting – a child who has a low threshold for response and who also is highly distractible might find it difficult to perform efficiently in a setting with high noise levels (e.g., a crowded home, a school room situated near the street in a busy urban area) when tasks necessitating concentration and/or attention (e.g., studying, taking an examination) are required.

Thomas and Chess (1977, 1980, 1981), J. Lerner (1983), and J. Lerner and R. Lerner (1983) believe that adaptive psychological and social functioning do not derive directly from either the nature of the person's characteristics per se or the nature of the demands of the contexts within which the person functions. Rather, if a person's characteristics match (or "fit") the demands of a particular setting, adaptive outcomes in that setting will accrue. Those people whose characteristics match most of their contexts should receive supportive or positive feedback and should show evidence of the most adaptive behavioral development. In turn, of course, mismatched people, whose characteristics are incongruent with one or more contexts, should experience maladaptive developmental outcomes.

In sum, the goodness-of-fit concept suggests that any given temperament attribute may or may not be associated with positive developmental outcomes; the relation depends on the way(s) in which the attribute meets the demands of the context. The same attribute (for example, low rhythmicity, or regularity, of biological functions) may be related to negative parent–child relations if the parent values or expects rhythmicity and/or if the parent's own behavioral style necessitates rhythmicity for positive interactions to occur. On the other hand, if the parent does not value or expect rhythmicity or if his or her own behavioral style does not necessitate it, low rhythmicity should not be related to negative parent–child relations; conceivably, it could be related, in a particular data set, to positive parent-child relations.

In short, unless one has knowledge of the demands of a particular setting, one cannot adequately predict or explain the absence or presence of a relation between an attribute of individuality and psychosocial functioning. It is the attribute–demand relation, the goodness of fit, and not the attribute alone, that should allow one to predict and explain psychosocial functioning in a given setting.

The major support for this goodness-of-fit model and for its synthesis with the circular functions model of Schneirla (1957) and the person–context relations model of R. Lerner (1979) and J. Lerner (1983), comes from research in the literature on temperament, a literature most influenced by the seminal work of Thomas and Chess (1977). *Temperament* is used here to refer not to the content of the behavioral repertoire (e.g., sleeping, eating, or toileting), but, following Thomas and Chess (1977), to *how* the person engages in those behaviors (e.g., sleeping or eating with rhythmicity or regularity). In other words, because all children engage in eating, sleeping, and toileting behaviors, the absence or presence of such behaviors would not differentiate among them, whereas whether these behaviors occur with regularity (e.g., rhythmically) or with a lot or a little intensity might serve to differentiate among them.

The New York Longitudinal Study

Data from the temperament research of Thomas, Chess, and their colleagues (e.g., Thomas, Chess, & Birch, 1968; Thomas et al., 1963) provide several instances of empirical support for the conceptual synthesis I am trying to make here among the three models noted in the preceding section. In their New York Longitudinal Study (NYLS) of the psychosocial significance of temperamental individuality, Thomas and Chess (Thomas & Chess, 1977; Thomas, Chess, Sillan, & Mendez, 1974) have prospectively studied, for over 25 years, a core sample of 133 white, middle-class, largely Jewish children of professional parents in New York City. In addition, a sample of 98 New York City Puerto Rican children of working-class parents have been followed for about 7 years. Each sample was studied from the first month of life onward. Although the distribution of temperamental attributes in the two samples was not different, the import of the attributes for psychosocial adjustment was quite disparate. Two examples are offered to illustrate this distinction.

Let us consider the impact of low regularity or rhythmicity of behavior, particularly in regard to sleep-wake cycles. The Puerto Rican parents studied by Thomas and Chess (Thomas & Chess, 1977; Thomas et al., 1974; see also Korn, 1978) were quite permissive. No demands in regard to rhythmicity of sleep were placed on the infant or child. Indeed, the parents allowed the child to go to sleep and awaken any time the child desired. The parents molded their schedule around the children. Thus, because parents were so accommodating, there were no problems of fit associated with an arrhythmic infant or child. Indeed, neither in infancy nor throughout the first five years of life did arrhythmicity predict adjustment problems. In this sample arrhythmicity remained continuous and independent of aptive implications for the child (Thomas et al., 1974).

In the white, middle-class families, however, strong demands for rhythmic sleep patterns were maintained. Thus, an arrhythmic child did not fit with parental demands, and consistent with the goodness-of-fit model, arrhythmicity was a major predictor of problem behaviors both in the infant years and across the first five years of life (Thomas et al., 1974). However, the parents in the white, middle-class sample took steps to change their arrhythmic children's sleep patterns; and since most of these arrhythmic children were also adaptable, low rhythmicity tended to be discontinuous for most children.

Thus, in the white middle-class sample, early infant arrhythmicity tended to be a problem during this time of life but proved to be neither continuous nor predictive of later problems of adjustment. In the Puerto Rican sample, infant arrhythmicity was not a problem during this time of life, but it was continuous and – because in the Puerto Rican context it was not involved in poor fit – it was not associated with adjustment problems in the first five years of life. However, to underscore the importance of considering the context of development in order to understand whether a behavioral attribute will show constancy or change from infancy onward, we should note that arrhythmicity did begin to predict adjustment problems for the Puerto Rican children when they entered the school system. Their lack of a regular sleep pattern interfered with their getting sufficient sleep to perform well in school and, in addition, often caused them to be late for school (Korn, 1978).

Thus, with hardly any pun intended, we have in the Puerto Rican data set an example of a type of "sleeper effect." Early (i.e., infant and later, child) measures of low rhythmicity predicted later life problems but did not relate to adjustment contemporaneously. Moreover, we see in the NYLS data an illustration of four points: (1) A given behavioral attribute may be either continuous or discontinuous; (2) this change may be promoted by the channeling effects of the socializing context – a point well made 20 years ago by Kagan and Moss (1962); (3) since infant attributes may therefore be either enduring or reversible, depending on their fit with the socializing, constraining, or enhancing context, we need to study the conditions that permit relations between organism and context to remain the same or change; and (4) whether any given infant attribute remains continuous or not, it may still have import for later life functioning, but such "connectivity" also depends critically on the changing context to which the developing organism must relate.

One final example from the NYLS data may be given in order to indicate how the differential demands of the white middle-class and the Puerto Rican working-class family contexts provided different presses for aptation. This example pertains to differences in the demands of the physical contexts of the families.

As noted by Thomas et al. (1974) as well as Korn (1978), overall there was a very low incidence of behavior problems in the Puerto Rican sample children in their first five years of life, especially when compared to the white, middle-class sample children. However, if a problem did arise at this time among the Puerto Rican sample it was most likely to be a problem of motor activity.

In the Puerto Rican sample the families usually had several children and lived in small apartments. Even average motor activity therefore tended to impinge on others in the setting. Moreover, even in the case of the children with high activity levels, the Puerto Rican parents were reluctant to let their children out of the apartment because of the dangers of playing on the streets of East Harlem. In the middle-class sample, however, the parents had the financial resources to provide large apartments or houses for their families. There were typically suitable play areas for the children both inside and outside the home. As a consequence, the presence of high activity levels in the homes of the middle-class sample did not cause the problems for interaction that they did in the Puerto Rican group. Thus, as Thomas et al. (1968, 1974) emphasize, the mismatch between temperamental attribute and physical environmental demand accounted for the group difference in the import of high activity level for the development of behavioral problems.

Data sets independent of the NYLS

There are other data pertinent to the goodness-of-fit model. In a series of cross-sectional studies in my laboratory, the use of the goodness-of-fit model has been supported among samples in the late childhood to late adolescent age range. J. Lerner (1983) used a version of the Dimensions of Temperament Survey (DOTS) to measure eighth-graders' temperaments. This instrument, developed by R. Lerner, Palermo, Spiro, and Nesselroade (1982), assesses multiple dimensions of temperament: activity level, rhythmicity, adaptability/approach–withdrawal, attention span–persistence/distractibility, and reactivity – the last being an attribute composed of items relating to threshold, activity level, and intensity. Lerner also assessed the demands for behavioral style in the classroom by each subject's classroom teacher and peer group. Those subjects whose temperaments best matched each set of demands had more favorable teacher ratings of adjustment and ability, better grades, more positive peer relations, fewer negative peer relations, and more positive self-esteem than did subjects whose temperaments were less well matched with either teacher or peer demands.

There is evidence that temperament–context fit also covaries with abilities, measured with standard psychometric instruments. That is, J. Lerner's (1983) study demonstrated a relation between peer and teacher ratings, on the one hand, and teacher-assigned grades and goodness of fit, on the other. However, no relation between academic abilities and fit was seen. Such a relation was found by J. Lerner, Lerner, and Zabski (in press), however. That is, for several dimensions measured by the DOTS, and most notably for reactivity, fourth-grade students whose self-rated temperament best fit teacher demands scored better on two standardized achievement tests – the Stanford Achievement Test for Reading and the Comprehensive Test of Basic Skills – then did less-well-fit children.

Moreover, in a study by Palermo (1982), fifth-graders' self-ratings of their temperament were found to be interchangeable with their mothers' ratings of their temperament in the prediction of teacher evaluations, peer relations, and parental identification of problem behaviors in the home. Again, better-fit children had more favorable scores on these measures than did less-well-fit children.

Most interestingly, in regard to the Palermo's data, the best predictors of *all* outcome measures – that is, of outcome measures derived from teacher, peer, and mother ratings – were fit scores computed between mother-rated temperament and teacher demands. In other words, Palermo's data provide the best indication that temperament is not a within-person phenomenon and especially not a maternal perception: Discrepancy scores derived from temperament rated by one source (mother) and demands derived from another independent source (teacher) not only were the best predictors of adjustment within the mother- and teacher-rated contexts but also within a third, independent (peer) context.

Palermo's (1982) study extended our research, beyond the school context, to the home setting. Kacerguis (1982) continued in this direction and focused on the pre- versus postpubescent daughter–mother dyad. Steinberg and Hill (1978) found that parental responses to their children differed in relation to the child's pubertal status; for example, more problematic relations existed in parent–child dyads including a postpubescent child. Such findings led Kacerguis to speculate that the source of parent–child conflict differs among pre- and postpubescent daughter–mother dyads – that is, that parents of prepubescents expect different behaviors of their children than do parents of postpubescents; as a consequence, Kacerguis predicted that to the extent that temperamental differences are involved in these different behavioral expectations, temperament should be differentially linked to parent–child conflict in the two puberty groups.

Studying a group of 53 prepubescent daughter-mother dyads and a group of 42 postpubescent daughter-mother dyads, Kacerguis (1982) obtained ratings by the mothers of the level of conflict in the parent–child relationship. In turn, through use of the DOTS, all adolescents rated their own temperaments. Kacerguis's predictions were confirmed. Among the prepubescent daughter–mother dyads higher levels of activity, rhythmicity, and reactivity were significantly related to higher levels of conflict (disattenuated r = .54, .79, and .81, respectively; p < .001 in all cases) and higher levels of attention and adaptability were significantly related to lower levels of conflict (disattenuated r = .66 and .70, respectively; p < .001 in both cases). However, the relations between temperament and parent–child conflict were markedly different among the postpubescent daughter-mother dyads. First, two significant reversals in direction of correlation occurred: Higher activity level and rhythmicity scores were associated in this group with lower conflict scores (disattenuated $r = .35$, $p < .05$, and $.43$, $p < .01$, respectively). Second, no significant correlations between either attention, adaptability, or reactivity and parent–child conflict were found, and all three of these correlations differed significantly from the corresponding ones among the prepubescent daughter–mother dyads ($p < .001$ in all cases).

Finally, in regard to a recent study in my laboratory, Windle and Lerner (in press) studied 153 late adolescent dating dyads, that is, college students engaged in exclusive dating relationships. Each dyad member's temperament and expectational demands for the partner's temperament were measured. Within-dyad temperament–temperament and expectation–expectation correlations were calculated for each of the five temperament attributes measured by the DOTS. Thus, the presence of fit with two aspects of a significant other were measured in this study; that is, behavioral style fit and expectational fit were assessed. These dating dyad correlations were compared to those that existed within 98 randomly formed dyads, that is, dyads formed by randomly pairing 98 nondating college males with 98 nondating college females. This comparison was made in order to assess if consistency between partners marks exclusive dating relationships or if any two people, no matter how paired, show a significant level of fit.

The results of these analyses indicate that within the dating dyads three of five temperament–temperament correlations (for adaptability, rhythmicity, and reactivity) and five of five demand–demand correlations were significant. In the "random dyads" only one of five temperament–temperament correlations (for rhythmicity) and none of the demand–demand correlations was significant. Moreover, the magnitudes of six of the eight significant correlations in the dating dyads were significantly greater than the corresponding correlation in the "random dyads." Thus, in this study, temperament–temperament fit and demand–demand fit seem to mark the relation between a late adolescent and a significant other in his or her social context. Such congruence appears to be absent among late adolescents not engaged in exclusive-dating or intimate relationships – a type of social relationship believed to be central to adequate psychosocial functioning during the late adolescent portion of life. This difference between the late adolescent groups suggests the importance of a goodness of fit between the person and his or her significant interpersonal context in adaptive functioning in this portion of the life span.

Conclusions

Along with the longitudinal analyses from the NYLS, the independent temperament research pertinent to the goodness-of-fit model provides initial support for the model and encourages its further use. Indeed, I believe an appropriate inference from this research is that at a given point in development neither children's attributes per se nor the demands of their setting per se are the key predictors of their aptive functioning. Instead, the *relation* between child and context seems most important in their peer, home, and school settings. Not meeting the demands of one's context (i.e., having a poor fit) is associated with adverse individual and interpersonal functioning. Accordingly, if differential goodness of fit does provide a basis for contrasting psychosocial functioning, then it is appropriate to initiate interventions aimed at enhancing fit.

The next section focuses on the relevance of the goodness-of-fit model for theory and practice in intervention.

Enhancing goodness of fit

Interventions aimed at enhancing goodness of fit, and thereby also enhancing the psychosocial functions that result from good fit, may be targeted at the level of the individual and/or at the level of the context. First, in regard to the context, one may attempt to modify one or more of the three demand domains noted earlier (attitudes, values, stereotypes of others; behavioral characteristics of others; physical characteristics of the setting). Among infants and very young children, for instance, such intervention targets may be the only ones available. Caregivers may have to be informed about the contextual nature of temperament and the role of fit with contextual demands in the infant's psychosocial development. Here the cognitive developmental level of the caregiver is itself an issue (Sameroff, 1975), since such educational interventions with the caregiver may be expected to vary in their success as a consequence of the caregiver's cognitive abilities to deal with the phenomena psychologists call "bidirectional influences," "goodness of fit," and "behavioral individuality." Thus, a complete intervention repertoire aimed at altering children's contexts affecting their caregivers might need to include behavior modification and parent education techniques as well as cognitive or cognitive–behavioral ones.

One might be prone to believe that to enhance fit among people in their aged years it would be necessary to rely on modification of contextual demands; however, there is an increasingly narrower but nevertheless still viable reservoir of plasticity in this phase of life – as we have noted in previous chapters in our discussion of the neuroanatomical concept of selective preservation (Greenough & Green, 1981) and of the life-span developmental psychological concept of selective optimization (Baltes & Baltes, 1980). Features of the particular aged population with which one is concerned (e.g., severely handicapped, institutionalized aged) as well as economic considerations may preclude any strategy other than a contextual one; nevertheless, the evidence pertinent to plasticity across the life span suggests that interventions aimed at the level of the individual are not precluded among the aged (Baltes & Baltes, 1980; Greenough & Green, 1981).

In turn, if one targets the individual for intervention, then one may focus one's efforts on altering the person's actions *in or on* the context, thereby changing the goodness of fit. This latter alternative is attractive for at least two reasons.

First, people have different levels of goodness of fit because of the differential impact of their characteristics on the context. Since it is the person, in all his or her individuality, that initiates the "circular functions" that help determine the level of fit, work focused on the individual is therefore directed at a key factor in the developmental process.

Second, with the individual playing so central a role in his or her own developmental processes, it is important to enhance the person's ability to regulate his or her own further development. If we changed a particular context for the person but did not give the person those behavioral and/or cognitive abilities needed to continue to alter *either self or context*, then it is unlikely the person would be able to exercise appropriate self-regulation when new contexts or demands were encountered. One cannot anticipate all the contexts and demands one may encounter in life; thus, it may be most efficient to focus one's intervention efforts on providing bases for the individual to change self *or* context. Moreover, a person's perceptual "filtering" of contextual demands is an important component of the ways in which demands operate; and this role played by the individual, as a key part of his or her own context, underscores the appropriateness of targeting interventions at the individual level of analysis. Thus, as I will now explain, by enhancing self-regulatory functions involved in allowing the person to become an active producer of his or her own development, one may be most appropriately and efficiently providing the means to enhance goodness of fit. Note, however, that I am *not* saying that one should eliminate individual differences in order to allow people to meet contextual demands. Rather, the goal is to provide the means by which people could alter themselves *or* the contextual demands imposed on them.

To begin this presentation, I should note that, by itself, the goodness-of-fit concept describes only the status of the relation between the person and his or her context at a particular point in time. However, a life-span developmental perspective emphasizes process and, as a consequence, a key concern in the application of the goodness-of-fit notion is the identification of the antecedent changes that resulted in a particular fit at a specific time and, in turn, specification of the consequences of this fit for later development. Only with such information can appropriate interventions be instituted. However, as emphasized by Kendall (1981), intervention should only proceed after necessary assessments are made; there are several cognitive and behavioral variables that would have to be assessed before one could intervene to enhance goodness of fit.

One would have to assess whether the person could appropriately evaluate (1) the demands of a particular context; (2) his or her stylistic attributes; and (3) the degree of match that exists between the two. In addition to these cognitive assessments, other cognitive and behavioral and skill assessments are necessary. One has to determine whether the person has the ability to select and gain access to those contexts with which there is a high probability of match and avoid those contexts where poor fit is likely. In addition, in those contexts that cannot easily be selected – for example, family of origin or assigned elementary school class – one has to assess whether the person has the knowledge and skills necessary either to change to fit the demands of the setting or alter the context to better fit the person's attributes (Mischel, 1977; Snyder, 1981). Moreover, in most contexts there will be multiple types of demands impinging on the person, and not all of them will provide identical demands. Thus, assessment needs to be made of whether the person can detect and evaluate such complexity. Furthermore, the absence or presence of skills in selecting those demands to which one will adapt (when all cannot be met) needs to be ascertained. Finally, it should be noted that in order for all these individual assessments to be useful, continuous assessments must be made of contextual demands. This need for monitoring both the individual and the context underscores the need for a multidisciplinary approach for the orientation I am advocating.

Appropriate individually oriented interventions based on such individual and contextual assessments might involve skill training, behavior modification, and/ or various cognitive–behavioral changes. The common goal of all procedures would be to enhance the person's ability for self-regulation and thereby increase the ability to actively enhance one's fit. Here it should be noted that J. Lerner (1983) found that the match scores between an adolescent's temperament and his or her perception of the demands placed on him or her were better predictors of adjustment than the match scores between temperament and actual demands; this finding suggests that such interventions may be derived from the work of Bandura on perceived self-efficacy (Bandura, 1978, 1980a, b).

Children who do not see themselves as efficacious in a particular setting will tend to withdraw from the situation, take a negative attitude toward the situation, and/or be less active in it (Bandura, 1980a, b). Bandura and Schunk (1981) report that such a style of behavior – one representative of those temperamental characteristics associated with problem behavior in the contexts of the middle-class family (Thomas et al., 1974) and of the school (Kohn, 1977) – was characteristic of elementary school students who were not doing well in mathematics. By withdrawing from the situation, the children were acting to enhance their own further failure, since by not actively or enthusiastically participating they were not exposing themselves to the experiences and practice opportunities necessary for success in mathematics.

Assessing children's perceptions of their efficacy before intervention revealed that they saw themselves (quite appropriately) as unable to do what was necessary for success in the situation. However, Bandura and Schunk found that enhancing the child's perceived self-efficacy engendered greater approach and activity. The child, now taking greater advantage of the learning experiences available in the context, eventually showed greater competence in mathematics.

The manipulation of self-efficacy is but one of the many behavioral or cognitive–behavioral strategies that may be adopted to enhance people's abilities to create better fits for themselves in their contexts. Still other strategies are outlined by Kendall (1981).

For example, Kendall describes an array of cognitive-behavioral interventions useful for teaching self-control in children. Children with problems in self-control are often referred to an interventionist because their characteristic style of behavior – a low threshold for response initiation (often described as "impulsive" behavior), high approach, and, often, high intensity responses and high activity levels – does not meet with the approval of parents and/or teachers. This lack of fit between their behavior and the values of others in their context often causes individual (e.g., academic achievement) problems as well as understandable ones in interpersonal relations.

Kendall notes that various training tasks may be initiated that involve, first, the acquisition of skills in verbal self-instruction. The therapist first teaches the use of self-instructions on simple academic tasks, gradually shifting to more difficult, impersonal problems, and finally to hypothetical interpersonal problems (Kendall, 1981, p. 58). For instance, in solving the simple academic tasks, verbal self-instruction training involves getting the child to ask "which one comes next" as he or she proceeds through each step of the problem. In addition to verbal self-instructions, Kendall (1981) describes various modeling, behavioral contingency management, role-playing, and self-evaluation procedures that are useful to institute in the elimination of self-control problems.

Conclusions

The work of Bandura (1980a, b) and Kendall (1981), among others (e.g., see Mischel, 1977; Snyder, 1981), suggests that an array of strategies exist for giving a person those cognitive and behavioral skills necessary to change self, context, or both. Thus, rather than being "passive recipients" of the fit immediately afforded them as a consequence of their temperamental characteristics, assessments and interventions associated with a process view of the goodness-of-fit concept can provide people with those abilities necessary to actively create a good fit for themselves and thus enhance their own further development.

A contextual view of temperament thus not only allows us to adequately understand how this facet of human individuality contributes to development, but in so doing it provides an excellent illustration of the way in which individuals themselves contribute to their own development. As such, it also offers an important example of the potential plasticity of human development and, as a consequence, of the potential for successfully intervening to enhance human life.

10 Conclusions: On the limits of plasticity and the plasticity of limits

The preceding chapters have, in my view, indicated that there is plasticity at each of the levels of analysis I have considered. Often, this plasticity derives from processes at one level of analysis influencing and being influenced by other levels' processes. Thus, key processes at any level may be appropriate targets of intervention as a consequence of this plasticity. And because of embeddedness of one level in another, one can modify processes at one level (e.g., cognitive–behavioral ones) to reach a target at another (e.g., those pertinent to neurotransmitters). Such reciprocity provides a compelling rationale of interdisciplinary research and intervention.

Accordingly, there is reason to be optimistic that in the future lie further paths to understanding how to better actualize humans' potential plasticity. But this optimism must be tempered by the recognition that along these paths lie two problematic sets of issues: First, throughout this book I have reviewed evidence that the organism's "reservoir" of plasticity decreases across life; that is, while plasticity is ubiquitous across life, the domains or band within which plasticity may be evidenced or actualized decrease. Second, there are several theoretical, substantive, and technological problems that must be resolved in order to further the ability of science to enhance human plasticity. These two sets of issues constitute significant limitations on both plasticity per se and knowledge about it. Let us treat each issue separately.

Plasticity as an ever-present but declining phenomenon

An organism's plasticity does not remain at a constant level across its life span. In Chapter 4, for example, we indicated that while evidence could be found for systematic neuroanatomical change across life (e.g., Cotman & Nieto-Sampedro, 1982; Greenough & Green, 1981; Lynch & Gall, 1979), the character of the changes could best be represented by the concept of "selective preservation" (Greenough & Green, 1981); that is, only some features of the neuronal architecture are preserved, and not all instances of an organism's neuroanatomy show

163

continued growth throughout life (see, e.g., Buell & Coleman, 1979). Similarly, on the human behavioral level, Baltes and Baltes (1980) have used the concept of "selective optimization" to indicate that in the aged years there remains only a subset of cognitive–behavioral functions that continue to remain available for change. In short, plasticity is not limitless, although it is ever-present in life.

We may introduce here several lines of work pertinent to this point. First, Mac Donald (1982), in a provocative essay integrating the concept of sensitive periods with the literature pertinent to early experience effects, makes several points consistent with the theme of plasticity as an ever-present but declining phenomenon.

Mac Donald's idea of *sensitive period* is best understood as a notion pertaining to the efficiency of environmental influences. The two key parameters of the concept are the age of the organism and the intensity of the environmental stimulus needed to modify the age effect. The concept of sensitive period therefore means that "deprivation or stimulation will be most efficient at producing effects at particular ages and that attempts at overriding these effects outside the sensitive period will tend to require relatively large investments of time or energy" (Mac Donald, 1982, p. 3).

For example, injection of testosterone propionate into newborn female mice results in greater masculinization than does injection at day 12 of life (Bronson & Desjardins, 1970); and if injection is delayed until day 30 a longer injection period is needed in order to obtain the same level of masculinization (Edwards, 1970). Similar findings were reported by Barraclough (1966). A progressively larger dose of testosterone propionate was needed to induce acyclicality in female rats at later ages. For instance, at 5 days of age, only 5 mg of testosterone propionate was needed to lower the proportion of cycling females to 56%. However, at 10 days of age, 1250 mg were needed to achieve a similar proportion. Thus, Mac Donald indicates, a larger dose or more intensive treatment is needed at later ages; that is, the organism is increasingly refractory to modification by environmental stimulation.

Mac Donald reviews other data on animals (e.g., Bateson, 1964; Hoffman & Rattner, 1973; Immelmann & Suomi, 1981) and humans (e.g., Flint, 1978; McKay et al., 1978) that support the above-described roles of the age and environmental-stimulus-intensity parameters of the sensitive periods notion. Together, these data suggest that while the organism can be changed across its life, it becomes increasingly more difficult to effect change; change requires a more intensive environmental stimulus. In other words, Mac Donald argues, plasticity is present across life, albeit to an increasingly narrower or more circumscribed extent, one described by the ideas of selective preservation (Greenough & Green, 1981) and selective optimization (Baltes & Baltes, 1980).

Implications for intervention

This idea of ubiquitous but declining plasticity has important implications for both intervention and social policy. The presence of plasticity across life might suggest to some that little investment in childhood is necessary; if one can correct undesired behaviors in later life, if effects of early experience can be counteracted, why be concerned with early life? However, the idea of plasticity that has found support in the research reviewed in this book – of ubiquitous but declining plasticity – suggests that the childhood years are indeed quite important.

Nevertheless, as Clarke and Clarke (1976) point out:

It is unclear whether the limits of personal change are the same throughout the period of development, or whether, as we rather suspect, they get progressively smaller as age increases and as personal characteristics in adolescence and young adult life begin to achieve an autonomy and self-perpetuation. This is our so-called "wedge" hypothesis, suggesting a greater potential responsiveness during early life and childhood at the "thick" end, trailing off to little responsiveness in adulthood, the "thin" end of the wedge. This hypothesis is difficult to test because children needing help either do or do not get it rather early in life; and the extreme cases of socialization can scarcely remain undetected beyond the age of school entry. Hence data on comparable environmental changes at very different ages hardly exist.

Similarly, Mac Donald (1982, pp. 56–57) concludes that

we have come a long way from supposing that behavior was absolutely fixed at an early age by genetic factors or, if indeed anyone did believe it, that after a sensitive period it was impossible to change behavior. Nevertheless, there are too many data showing otherwise to believe in the infinite plasticity of human or animal behavior. This fact does not of course prevent us from finding ways to intervene with individuals who have suffered early environmental insults. Indeed the theory of sensitive periods suggests that the intensity of an ecologically appropriate stimulus can, at least up to a point, overcome the organism's declining plasticity. The fact of declining plasticity merely indicates what we already know, that successful interventions are not easily come by.

Plasticity and constancy in development

Of course, the fact that one does not see a change over time in behavior cannot be taken as proof of the absence of plasticity (Mac Donald, 1982). Constancy in the individual can be due to consistency in the demands or constraints of the environment within which the individual is functioning and to which the individual must adapt (see Wohlwill, 1980). In addition, with regard to data she reviewed Clarke (1982, p. 73) indicates that "there is substantial reason to postulate a biological trajectory from which individuals may deviate when environmental deprivation is severe, but to which they will return when these stresses are removed or significantly diminished," and that there is also a social trajectory determined within broad limits by accident of birth and alterable by chance or design. Normally the two trajectors are interlocking, but in studies of deviant development they may not be so. The two trajectories are helpful conceptually in explaining apparently spontaneous recovery from deprivation. The idea is derived from the work of the British geneticist, Waddington (1957, 1966), who has drawn attention to a "self-righting tendency" which pushes deprived children towards normality whenever circumstances allow.

In addition, and especially among humans, developing individuals' progressive ability to be competent in self-regulation means that individuals become better able to self-select and shape the context within which they interact and thereby produce or maintain their constancy (R. Lerner, 1982; R. Lerner & Busch-Rossnagel, 1981; Mischel, 1977; Synder, 1981). Given that contextual presses could be changing while such individual production processes are occurring, the maintenance of individual constancy in such a case would be evidence of con-siderable flexibility on the part of the individual.

Unfortunately, however, neither the environmental nor the individual sources of constancy have been well studied (Mac Donald, 1982; Wohlwill, 1980). Cairns and Hood (1983), however, discuss five factors that give rise to individual continuity in development. They note that, first, individual-specific biological variables may contribute to continuity in an individual's behavior. Such variables include genetic processes that might endure over several developmental periods, hormonal processes, and morphology. However, they caution that

biological factors are rarely translated directly into differences in social interaction patterns. The *linkages* between psychobiological processes and social behavior patterns *need to be examined at each of the several points in ontogeny*. It cannot be safely assumed that biological or genetic-based differences persist, unmodified by social encounters or interchanges in which the individual engages. (Cairns & Hood, 1983, p. 8; italics added)

The second factor that Cairns and Hood identify as potentially contributing to the continuity of behavior is the social network in which development occurs; they believe that, if all other factors are equal, similarities in behavior from one time to the next will be greatest when this social network remains constant. This may be especially true of insulated people (Wahler, 1980). The third factor Cairns and Hood identify is behavioral consolidation, based on social learning, of interactional learning experiences.

The fourth and fifth factors noted by Cairns and Hood are ones we have seen suggested before. "Social evocation and mutual control" allow individuals to contribute to the continuity of their own behavior by virtue of their being involved in a "circular function" (Schneirla, 1957). That is, by virtue of their physical and behavioral characteristics of individuality, people evoke differential reactions in others, reactions that involve (1) classification of the person–stimulus into categories (e.g., attractive, overweight, male, black); and (2) category-specific feedback to the person (R. Lerner, 1976; see too Kendall, Lerner, & Craighead, in press). Cairns and Hood note that "to the extent that some stimulus properties of the individual remain relatively constant over time, the social actions contingent upon the actions of others may themselves remain relatively similar" (p. 10).

Finally, Cairns and Hood note that individuals may actively promote their own continuity. Especially as self-regulatory competency increases, individuals make choices, exhibit preferences, and take actions that preserve their social network and their social relations and that maintain their environmental setting (cf. Kendall et al., in press; Mischel, 1977; Snyder, 1981).

In sum, Cairns and Hood observe that there are several processes that may maintain constancy in an organism's behavior and that none of these pertains to the lasting or constraining effects of early experience or directly speaks to the level of plasticity typical of organisms across their development. In other words, the presence of constancy across development is not, in and of itself, evidence against (or for) the view that organisms remain plastic across life (Cairns & Hood, 1983; see also Mac Donald, 1982; Wohlwill, 1980).

Conclusions

Not only does plasticity represent across life a ubiquitous but declining phenomenon; also, because an instance of plasticity may involve the organism's actively and creatively maintaining a context within which it can remain constant, the presence of plasticity may be difficult to verify. Indeed, in this view, the presence of constancy may be an index of plasticity. Thus, the outcomes of effects of plasticity may be difficult to disentangle from other phenomena leading to constancy (or change).

To aid in this process of separation a clear specification of the parameters of plasticity would be useful. But attempts to make such specification are limited by the second set of issues I noted at the outset of this chapter, those dealing with theoretical, substantive, and technological problems involved in our knowledge about plasticity. Let us now consider these issues.

Parameters of plasticity

First, substantively, we must recognize that despite the amount of evidence that exists for human plasticity, we still cannot answer several fundamental questions about the parameters of plasticity. Are processes at different levels of analysis differentially plastic? Are different targets within levels differentially flexible? For example, while recombinant DNA technology has put us on the threshold of gene therapy, it may still be the case that selected features of our genotype (e.g., the number of chromosomes we possess) cannot be altered (without, at least, severely damaging our organismic integrity) no matter what the nature of organism–context relations may be. On the other hand, more molar, behavioral features of functioning (e.g., those at the cognitive–behavioral level) may not present such restrictions. For instance, are there limits to the number of languages a person can learn to speak, or the number of names of people a person may know? No current evidence indicates that such limits exist.

In addition to not fully knowing the limits of plasticity that may currently characterize levels of analysis, we do not know what future substantive and technological advances may imply for the character of these limits. For example, the geneticist D. D. Brown (1981) notes that just a few years ago we could not even imagine how we could ever isolate a gene. Yet as geneticist Paul Berg (1981) notes, not only is such isolation today quite routine, but the growth in the application of recombinant DNA methods has been truly explosive. For instance, he observes that

molecular cloning provides the means to solve the organization and detailed molecular structure of extended regions of chromosomes and eventually the entire genome, including man. Already, investigators have isolated a number of mammalian and human genes, and in some instances determined their chromosomal arrangement and even their detailed nucleotide sequence. (P. 302)

Thus, if we take the idea of probabilistic epigenesis seriously, and if we recognize that science and technology represent natural parts of the human ecology, then we cannot anticipate where future scientific advances may lead. As a consequence, current limits of plasticity are not necessarily future ones. These limits are themselves plastic and will likely become increasingly broader in ways that, for some of us, are beyond our imagination.

As Toulmin (1981, p. 261) has put the issue:

As for the possibilities open to future, more complex cultures, there too we must be prepared to speculate open-mindedly. There, perhaps, people generally will take pride in having overcome the "illusions" of material conservation and Euclidean space alike, and may come to talk about everyday material objects with the same conceptual sophistication we ourselves display toward such un-everyday things as electrons.

But recognition that the limits of plasticity can change over time raises a developmental issue. The actualization of plasticity of course involves change, and change can only be identified over time. Numerous questions exist about the rates of change of plastic processes at the several levels of analysis that transact to provide the bases of behavior. First, it is clear that there is a "nonequivalent temporal metric" across the various levels of analysis (R. Lerner, Skinner, & Sorell, 1980) involved in person–context transactions. That is, as was illustrated in Figure 2 (Chapter 8), all levels of the context change over time; but time may not have an identical meaning at all the levels. One way to understand this is to note that the smallest meaningful division of time to detect change differs among levels. If time is one's "X axis," with the "Y axis" reflecting levels of one's target process, then sensible X-axis divisions to detect infant neuromuscular changes may be as large as weeks, whereas sensible X-axis divisions to detect neurotransmitter changes may be as small as minutes (Hosobuchi et al., 1982). However, the smallest sensible division to detect social change may be a year. In addition, even within a given level, time may not have an equivalent meaning at different points in development. For example, on the level of the individual, a 1-year separation between birthdays may seem to a 5-year-old to be a vast length of time; to someone experiencing his or her 39th birthday the 1-year period until the 40th birthday may seem quite short; and to an 85-year old, having to wait for 1 year for some important event may again seem quite long.

Implications for intervention

The import of the nonequivalent temporal metric is that it may be difficult to detect, on one level, the influence of changes promoted on another level; for example, a change on the biological level (e.g., as promoted through better nutritional programs for children) may be difficult to detect on the societal level. Indeed, an attempt to verify the existence of such an influence may require taking a long-term, perhaps intergenerational, perspective (Sarason, 1973); or in a within-cohort analysis, it may be possible to assess only interindividual differences in intraindividual change, and not intraindividual change itself. Complicating this issue is that even though the effects of a biological intervention on society may take a long time to detect, there is not necessarily symmetry of influence. That is, "upper-level" societal alteration and social change may impact quite visibly and relatively rapidly on "lower-level" individual and biological processes, but not vice versa. For example, changes in federal government funding programs, such as for school lunch programs for the poor, aid to dependent mothers, or Medicare and Medicaid, can impact relatively quickly on health, cognitive, and familial functioning variables associated with an individual.

The issues of the nonequivalent temporal metric and asymmetry of interlevel influences can be seen to lead to other ones. First, given different levels' rates of change, one needs to know how processes at different levels connect to one another: How do interlevel influences occur? The "goodness–of–fit" concept, discussed in the preceding chapter, is an illustration of an attempt to answer this question insofar as the individual and his or her immediate social context is concerned. However, there are perhaps an infinite number of possible interlevel relations that may occur; at this writing, we simply have not devoted enough thought and empirical energies to their investigation.

In turn, the issue of symmetry of interlevel influence raises similarly largely unaddressed concerns about efficiency and about cost/benefit ratios. To reach a target at an individual's cognitive–behavioral level – for example, the target of academic achievement – is it most efficient to institute a "bottom-up strategy" (e.g., at the biological level), a "parallel-level" strategy (e.g., by cognitive–behavioral means), or a "top-down" strategy (by instituting or changing social programs)? Which strategy leads to the most benefits, relative to economic, social, and personal costs? Simply, we do not know answers to these questions for very many of the potential targets of intervention.

Moreover, a decision about the level of analysis on which to focus one's intervention efforts is complicated by the fact that all levels of analysis are developing, are changing over time. While this feature of the human condition permits both concurrent and historical interventions, it again raises questions of efficiency and cost/benefit ratios. For example, when during the life span is it best to intervene to optimize a particular target process (and, of course, on what level is it best to focus one's efforts)? Are periods of developmental transition (e.g., puberty, retirement), or periods of relatively more stability, better times within which to focus one's efforts? Moreover, do some intervention goals – for example, the elimination of fetal alcohol syndrome (FAS) (Streissguth et al., 1980) – require an intergenerational–developmental rather than an ontogenetic–developmental approach? In the case of FAS, for instance, may not it be of more benefit to intervene with women before they become pregnant? Developmental intervention issues such as these have received relatively little attention.

A final, relatively ignored area relevant here relates to the issues of direct and indirect intervention effects and of planned and unplanned effects. If an individual's plasticity both derives from and contributes to interrelated levels of analysis, then one must anticipate that actualizing the potential for plasticity at any one level will influence changes among other variables, both at that and at other levels. From this perspective, one should always expect that any direct and/or intended effect of intervention will have indirect and often unintended consequences (Willems, 1973). Indeed, one may obtain desired indirect effects and/or unintended consequences of intervention even though one's planned, intended effects did not materialize.

An excellent illustration of how interventions may lead to unplanned outcomes that may be indirectly related to the target variable is found in the research reported by Lazar et al. (1982). These authors report the results of a multisample secondary analysis assessing the long-term effects of early childhood education experiences on children from low-income families, children who had been part of one of 12 independently designed and implemented infant and preschool programs begun in the 1960s. In 1976 a collaborative follow-up was conducted of the original subjects, who were ages 9 to 19 years at the time. With attrition analyses indicating essentially random attrition, Lazer et al. concluded that there were long-lasting effects of early education programs for children from low-income families in four areas:

1. Children in these programs were more likely to meet their schools' basic requirements, less likely to be assigned to special education classes, and less likely to be retained in grade than were controls.
2. Children in these programs did better than controls on the Stanford–Binet intelligence test for several years after the program had ended. However, there was no evidence that program participation raised IQ scores.

Indeed, Ramey (1982) points out that

none of the projects succeeded in developing children who, as a group, were significantly above average intellectually or, presumably, academically. In fact, the mean IQ performance at follow-up for the children from the four projects having more nearly randomized designs is approximately one standard deviation below the national average, for both program and control children. Clearly, then, this represents a group of children who are likely to experience major hardships in an increasingly technological and sophisticated culture. That these results obtained in spite of the efforts of some of our leading social scientists and educators testifies to the difficult and complex set of conditions associated with lower socioeconomic status in this country.

3. Nevertheless, despite the failure to boost IQ scores, children who had been in the program were, when tested in 1976, more likely than controls to give achievement-related reasons for being proud of themselves.
4. Finally, program participation altered children's familial context; that is, participation influenced mothers' attitudes concerning school performance and their vocational aspirations for their children.

Acknowledging the possibility of unplanned and/or indirect consequences of interventions leads to two points. First, interventions should not be initiated without some conceptual or theoretical analysis of the potential indirect and unintended consequences. For instance, changing a spouse's assertiveness may be the direct intended effect of a cognitive–behavior therapist's efforts, but the changed assertiveness might lead to a diminution of marital quality, even divorce. Such indirect effects might have been unintended by the therapist and undesired by either therapist or client. Thus, my view is that one must think quite seriously about the broader, contextual effects of intervention efforts. Clearly, a contextual, life-span perspective like the one I have been using throughout this book would be of use in this regard. It would sensitize one to the general possibility of, and perhaps some specific instances of, indirect effects of intervention efforts. Such reflection will be useful in several ways, a major one being that undesirable indirect effects may be anticipated; if so, then the issue of cost/benefit ratios can be engaged before intervention begins.

Of course, the fact that undesired effects may arise from intervention efforts again raises a point that I have emphasized throughout this book – that plasticity is a ''double-edged sword'': Plasticity permits planned interventions to enhance the human condition, but also allows aversive unintended or indirect effects.

Sigman (1982), while making similar points about the double-edged nature of plasticity and the import of this nature for intervention, makes an additional, provocative point linking plasticity and intervention with life-span development. If the system remains open to interventions at one point in time, then it may similarly remain open throughout life; as such, one cannot expect a planned intervention to effect permanent change when, after the intervention is completed, life circumstances may impose numerous potentially countervailing, unplanned interventions. As a consequence, one must take a life-span perspective toward intervention. As Sigman (1982, p. 112) indicates:

> Finally, the evidence on plasticity in childhood and adult years has an additional implication for intervention. Almost all research and clinical studies agree that there is significant plasticity in behavior at all ages. While the debate continues as to whether early plasticity is greater than that observed later in life, the capacity for recovery remains at all ages. This observation suggests that remediation can be attempted at all ages. If intervention is not planned in the early years, clinical treatment can be initiated in later childhood and adolescence.
>
> On the other hand, the evidence of continued plasticity cuts both ways. ... Our awareness of the individual's continued responsiveness to the environment should make us more conservative in our expectation that intervention for a brief period in early infancy will have long-term effects over time. We cannot anticipate that early intervention will be an inoculation against the trauma of all future environments. Although change brought about in the family may have more lasting effects, the family is also responsive to the greater milieu. With both child and family showing significant plasticity, intervention efforts must be sustained. Only by improving living and rearing conditions throughout childhood can we expect to promote continual developmental progress at the optimal level.

Finally, it should be noted here that the double-edged nature of plasticity, and the import of this nature for intervention, is complicated when we recall that, as a consequence of embeddedness, failure to intervene – to alter the context of life – is itself an intervention (i.e., it allows the individual or context to remain on a trajectory from which it might have diverged if one had acted). Thus, one must assess the cost/benefit ratio not only of one's actions, but too of one's failure to act. Such decisions rest on one's values.

Values and intervention

What is enhancement and how does one choose a target to enhance? On what do we base our decisions about whether the potential gains of our action (or inaction) outweigh the potential costs? Given human plasticity, in what direction do we attempt to move people in order to optimize their lives? Clearly, the behaviors, social institutions, and social functions one values critically affect one's answers to these questions.

For example, does enhancement mean increasing people's intelligence? Does it involve increasing personal freedom and/or individuality, or does it pertain to building group cohesiveness and respect for the collective nature of human life? Is enhancement the creation of equality between the sexes or among the races, or is it inculcating in all a respect for individual differences in abilities or life styles?

In my view, there are no right or wrong answers to these questions. What one sees as enhancement, another might see as deterioration; a target one person regards as valuable to enhance another might regard as irrelevant for bettering the human condition. The direction in which I might choose to move society might be viewed by another as unwise and perhaps dangerous. In other words, *any* intervention effort rests on values, and we should not expect to win un-equivocal respect and approval for our enhancement efforts, since value differ-ences pervade our society. The court decisions that mandated bussing to increase school integration were seen by some as a useful intervention aimed at bettering the quality of our society; by others the decisions were viewed as unjust and unfair infringements upon family and community life – for example, upon the rights of parents to give their children the opportunity to attend schools close to home.

The ubiquitous role of values in intervention – and I might add, in science as well – should not be ignored. One should be aware of, and attempt to be articulate and communicative about, the values one is promoting by one's intervention and about the potential risks that go along with the benefits one envisions. Moreover, in the process of making decisions about whether a particular inter-vention should be instituted, one should take into account the perspective of the human targets of one's efforts. Indeed, by actively integrating the people one is attempting to enhance into one's plans and procedures, one may take advantage of the active character of human functioning. One may thereby engage people's self-regulatory abilities and, as a consequence, facilitate their active contribution to their own plastic behavioral development (R. Lerner, 1982; R. Lerner & Busch-Rossnagel, 1981).

Conclusions

Any one problem of human development not only can and probably does derive from multiple sources but, because of the nature of the person's plasticity, the problem may be approached by a variety of intervention strategies associated with multiple levels of analysis. Both the assessment and intervention tasks, as well as the basic research underlying these endeavors, called for by a life-span perspective and necessitated by the nature of human plasticity, are multivariate ones. As noted, however, it is not probable that either we or our students can all become, by ourselves, multivariate researchers and multidisciplinary intervenors.

Yet we can, and indeed should, become aware of the complex, dynamic interactions among levels of analysis that both result from and lead to plasticity in human development. We should then build into our professional agendas collaboration that takes us beyond the disciplinary isolationism that has traditionally characterized most of academe.

All of us are concerned with the same organism. The nature of that organism requires us not only to do more science, but to do science differently. I am convinced that endeavors such as I have described and proposed can profoundly enhance human life.

References

Abel, E. L., Busch, R., & Dintcheff, B. A. 1981. Exposure of rats in utero alters drug sensitivity in adulthood. *Science, 212*, 1531–3.

Abravanel, E. 1968. The development of intersensory patterning with regard to selected spatial dimensions. *Monographs of the Society for Research in Child Development, 33* (2, No. 118).

Akil, H., Mayer, D. J., & Liebeskind, J. C. 1976. Reduction of stimulation-produced analgesia by the narcotic antagonist, naloxone. *Science, 191*, 961–2.

Anderson, P. W. 1972. More is different. *Science, 177*, 393–6.

Anderson, W. F. 1982. Technical and medical state-of-the art of gene therapy in human adults and embryos. *Abstracts of Papers of the 148th National Meeting of the American Association for the Advancement of Science* (abstract).

Anderson, W. F., & Diacumakos, E. G. 1981. Genetic engineering in mammalian cells. *Scientific American, 245*, 106–21.

Anderson, W. F., & Fletcher, J. C. 1980. Gene therapy in human beings: When is it ethical to begin? *New England Journal of Medicine, 303*, 1293–7.

Archer, S. M., Dubin, M. W., & Stark, L. A. 1982. Abnormal development of kitten retino-geniculate connectivity in the absence of action potentials. *Science, 217*, 743–5.

Arendash, G. W., & Gorski, R. A. 1982. Enhancement of sexual behavior in female rats by neonatal transplantation of brain tissue from males. *Science, 217*, 1276–8.

Bakan, D. 1966. *The duality of human existence*. Chicago: Rand McNally.

Baldwin, J. M. 1897. *Mental development in the child and the race*. New York: Macmillan.

Baldwin, J. M., & Poulton, E. B. 1902. Plasticity. In J. M. Baldwin (Ed.), *Dictionary of philosophy and psychology* (Vol. 2). New York: Peter Smith.

Baltes, P. B. 1968. Longitudinal and cross-sectional sequences in the study of age and generation effects. *Human Development, 11*, 145–71.

Baltes, P. B. (Ed.). 1978. *Life-span development and behavior* (Vol. 1). New York: Academic Press.

Baltes, P. B. 1979a. Life-span developmental psychology: Some converging observations on history and theory. In P. B. Baltes & O. G. Brim, Jr. (Eds.), *Life-span development and behavior* (Vol. 2). New York: Academic Press.

Baltes, P. B. 1979b. On the potential and limits of child development: Life-span developmental perspectives. *Newsletter of the Society for Research in Child Development*, Summer, 1–4.

Baltes, P. B., Baltes, M. M., & Reinert, G. 1970. The relationship between time of measurement and age in cognitive development of children: An application of cross-sectional sequences. *Human Development, 13*, 258–68.

Baltes, P. B., & Baltes, M. M. 1980. Plasticity and variability in psychological aging: Methodological and theoretical issues. In G. E. Gurski (Ed.), *Determining the effects of aging on the central nervous system*. Berlin: Schering AG (Oraniendruck).

175

Baltes, P. B., & Brim, O. G., Jr., (Eds.). 1979. *Life-span development and behavior* (Vol. 2). New York: Academic Press.

Baltes, P. B., & Brim, O. G., Jr., (Eds.). 1980. *Life-span development and behavior* (Vol. 3). New York: Academic Press.

Baltes, P. B., & Brim, O. G., Jr., (Eds.). 1981. *Life-span development and behavior* (Vol. 4). New York: Academic Press.

Baltes, P. B., Cornelius, S. W., & Nesselroade, J. R. 1977. Cohort effects in behavioral development: Theoretical and methodological perspectives. In W. A. Collins (Ed.), *Minnesota symposia on child psychology* (Vol. II). New York: Thomas Crowell.

Baltes, P. B., & Danish, S. J. 1980. Intervention in life-span development and aging: Issues and concepts. In R. R. Turner & H. W. Reese (Eds.). *Life-span developmental psychology: Intervention*. New York: Academic Press.

Baltes, P. B., Dittmann-Kohli, F., & Dixon, R. A. In press. New perspectives on the development of intelligence in adulthood: Toward a dual-process conception and a model of selective optimization with compensation. In P. B. Baltes & O. G. Brim, Jr. (Eds.), *Life-span development and behavior* (Vol. 6). New York: Academic Press.

Baltes, P. B., & Nesselroade, J. R. 1973. The developmental analysis of individual differences on multiple measures. In J. R. Nesselroade & H. W. Reese (Eds.), *Life-span developmental psychology: Methodological issues*. New York: Academic Press.

Baltes, P. B., Reese, H. W., & Lipsitt, L. P. 1980. Life-span developmental psychology. *Annual Review of Psychology, 31*, 65–110.

Baltes, P. B., Reese, H. W., & Nesselroade, J. R. 1977. *Life-span developmental psychology: Introduction to research methods*. Monterey, Calif.: Brooks/Cole.

Baltes, P. B., & Schaie, K. W. (Eds.). 1973. *Life-span developmental psychology: Personality and socialization*. New York: Academic Press.

Baltes, P. B., & Schaie, K. W. 1974. The myth of the twilight years. *Psychology Today, 7*, 35–40.

Baltes, P. B., & Schaie, K. W. 1976. On the plasticity of intelligence in adulthood and old age: Where Horn and Donaldson fail. *American Psychologist, 31*, 720–5.

Baltes, P. B., & Willis, S. L. 1981. Plasticity and enhancement of intellectual functioning in old age: Penn State's Adult Development and Enrichment Project (ADEPT). In F. I. M. Craik & S. E. Trehub (Eds.), *Aging and cognitive processes*. New York: Plenum Press.

Baltes, P. B., & Willis, S. L. 1982. Enhancement (plasticity) of intellectual functioning in old age: Penn State's Adult Development and Enrichment Project (ADEPT). In F. I. M. Craik & S. E. Trehub (Eds.), *Aging and cognitive processes*. New York: Plenum.

Bandura, A. 1965. Influence of models' reinforcement contingencies on the acquisition of imitative responses. *Journal of Personality and Social Psychology, 1*, 589–95.

Bandura, A. 1971. *Social learning theory*. Morristown, N.J.: General Learning Press.

Bandura, A. 1977. *Social learning theory*. Englewood Cliffs, N.J.: Prentice-Hall.

Bandura, A. 1978. The self system in reciprocal determinism. *American Psychologist, 33*, 344–58.

Bandura, A. 1980a. Self-referent thought: A developmental analysis of self-efficacy. In J. H. Flavell & L. D. Ross (Eds.), *Cognitive social development: Frontiers and possible futures*. New York: Cambridge University Press.

Bandura, A. 1980b. The self and mechanisms of agency. In J. Suls (Ed.), *Social psychological perspectives on the self*. Hillsdale, N.J.: Erlbaum.

Bandura, A. 1982. The psychology of chance encounters and life paths. *American Psychologist, 37*, 747–55.

Bandura, A., & Schunk, D. H. 1981. Cultivating competence, self-efficacy, and intrinsic interest through proximal self-motivation. *Journal of Personality and Social Psychology, 41*, 586–98.

Barbeau, A., Growdon, J. H., & Wurtman, R. J. (Eds.). 1979. *Nutrition and the brain*, Vol. 5: *Choline and lecithin in brain disorders*. New York: Raven Press.

Barchas, J. D., & Sullivan, S. 1982. Opioid peptides as neuroregulators: Potential areas for the study of genetic-behavioral mechanisms. *Behavior Genetics, 12,* 69–91.

Barraclough, C. A. 1966. Modifications of CNS regulation of reproduction after exposure of pre-pubertal rats to steroid hormones. *Recent Progress in Hormone Research, 22,* 503–39.

Bartus, R. T., Dean, R. L., Beer, B., & Lippa, A. S. 1982. The cholinergic hypothesis of geriatric memory dysfunction. *Science, 217,* 408–17.

Bates, J. E. 1980. The concept of difficult temperament. *Merrill–Palmer Quarterly, 26,* 299–319.

Bateson, P. P. G. 1964. Effects of similarity between rearing and testing conditions on chicks' following and avoiding responses. *Journal of Comparative and Physiological Psychology, 57,* 100–3.

Bayer, S. A., Yackel, J. W., & Puri, P. S. 1982. Neurons in the rat dentate gyrus granular layer substantially increase during juvenile and adult life. *Science, 216,* 890–2.

Baumrind, D. 1978. A dialectical materialist's perspective on knowing social reality. *New Directions for Child Development, 2,* 61–82.

Beatty, W. W. 1982. Peptides: Will they lead us to the engram? *Contemporary Psychology, 27,* 727–8.

Bell, R. Q. 1968. A reinterpretation of the direction of effects in studies of socialization. *Psychological Review, 75,* 81–95.

Bell, R. Q. 1974. Contributions of human infants to caregiving and social interaction. In M. Lewis & L. A. Rosenblum (Eds.), *The effect of the infant on its caregiver.* New York: Wiley.

Belsky, J. 1981. Early human experience: A family perspective. *Developmental Psychology, 17,* 3–23.

Belsky, J. In press. The determinants of parenting: A process model. *Child Development.*

Bengston, V. L., & Kuypers, J. A. 1971. Generational differences and the developmental stake. *Aging and Human Development, 2,* 249–60.

Bengtson, V. L., & Troll, L. 1978. Youth and their parents: Feedback and intergenerational influence in socialization. In R. M. Lerner & G. B. Spanier (Eds.), *Child influences on marital and family interaction: A life-span perspective.* New York: Academic Press.

Benveniste, R. E., & Todaro, G. J. 1982. Gene transfer between eukaryotes. *Science, 217,* 1202.

Berg, P. 1981. Dissections and reconstructions of genes and chromosomes. *Science, 213,* 296–303.

Berscheid, E., & Walster, E. 1974. Physical attractiveness. In L. Berkowitz (Ed.), *Advances in experimental social psychology.* New York: Academic Press.

Bertolini, A., & Poggioli, R. 1981. Chloramphenicol administration during brain development: Impairment of avoidance learning in adulthood. *Science, 213,* 238–9.

Bijou, S. W. 1976. *Child development: The basic stage of early childhood.* Englewood Cliffs, N.J.: Prentice-Hall.

Birch, H. G., & Lefford, A. 1963. Intersensory development in children. *Monographs of the Society for Research in Child Development, 28* (5, Serial No. 89).

Birch, H. G., & Lefford, A. 1967. Visual differentiation, intersensory integration, and voluntary motor control. *Monographs of the Society for Research in Child Development, 32* (2, No. 110).

Black, J. B. 1982. Stages of neurotransmitter development in autonomic neurons. *Science, 215,* 1198–204.

Block, J. 1982. Assimilation, accommodation, and the dynamics of personality development. *Child Development, 53,* 281–95.

Block, J. H. 1973. Conceptions of sex roles: Some cross-cultural and longitudinal perspectives. *American Psychologist, 28,* 512–26.

Block, J. H., & Block, J. 1980. The role of ego-control and ego-resiliency in the organization of behavior. In W. A. Collins (Ed.), *Minnesota Symposia on child psychology* (Vol. 13). Hillsdale, N.J.: Erlbaum.

Bock, W. 1967. The use of adaptive characters in avian classification. *Proceedings of the XIV International Ornithology Congress.*

Bock, W. 1979. A synthetic explanation of macroevolutionary change – a reductionistic approach. *Bulletin of the Carnegie Museum of Natural History, 13*, 20–69.

Bock, W. J. 1980. The definition and recognition of biological adaptation. *American Zoologist, 20*, 217–27.

Bodmer, W. F., & Cavalli-Sforza, L. L. 1976. *Genetics, evolution, and man*. San Francisco: Freeman.

Bolles, R. C., & Fanselow, M. S. 1982. Endorphins and behavior. *Annual Review of Psychology, 33*, 87–101.

Bondareff, W. 1981. The neurobiological basis of age-related changes in neuronal connectivity. In J. L. McGaugh, J. G. March, & S. B. Kiesler (Eds.), *Aging: Biology and Behavior*. New York: Academic Press.

Bondareff, W., & Geinisman, Y. 1976. Loss of synapses in the dentate gyrus of the senescent rat. *American Journal of Anatomy, 145*, 129–36.

Boothe, R. G., Greenough, W. T., Lund, J. S., & Wrege, K. 1979. A quantitative investigation of spine and dendritic development of neurons in visual cortex (area 17) of Macaca nemestrina monkeys. *Journal of Comparative Neurology, 186*, 473–90.

Bregman, B. S., & Goldberger, M. E. 1982. Anatomical plasticity and sparing of function after spinal cord damage in neonatal cats. *Science, 217*, 553–5.

Brent, S. B. 1978a. Individual specialization, collective adaptation and rate of environment change. *Human Development, 21*, 21–33.

Brent, S. B. 1978b. Prigogine's model for self-organization in nonequilibrium systems: Its relevance for developmental psychology. *Human Development, 21*, 374–87.

Brent, S. B. In press. *Psychological and social structure: Their organization, activity, and development*. New York: Erlbaum.

Bridges, R. S., & Grimm, C. T. 1982. Reversal of morphine disruption of maternal behavior by concurrent treatment with the opiate antagonist naloxone. *Science, 218*, 166–8.

Brim, O. G., Jr. 1968. Adult socialization. In J. A. Clausen (Ed.), *Socialization and society*. Boston: Little, Brown.

Brim, O. G., Jr. 1982. Some implications for child policy of life-span development research. *Social Policy Newsletter*, Spring, 4.

Brim, O. G., Jr., & Kagan, J. 1980. Constancy and change: A view of the issues. In O. G. Brim, Jr., & J. Kagan (Eds.), *Constancy and change in human development*. Cambridge: Harvard University Press.

Brim, O. G., Jr., & Ryff, C. D. 1980. On the properties of life events. In P. B. Baltes & O. G. Brim, Jr. (Eds.), *Life-span development and behavior* (Vol. 3). New York: Academic Press.

Brim, O. G., Jr., & Wheeler, S. 1966. *Socialization after childhood: Two essays*. New York: Wiley.

Bronfenbrenner, U. 1977. Toward an experimental ecology of human development. *American Psychologist, 32*, 513–31.

Bronfenbrenner, U. 1979. *The ecology of human development*. Cambridge: Harvard University Press.

Bronson, F. H., & Desjardins, C. 1970. Neonatal androgen and adult aggressiveness in female mice. *General and Comparative Endocrinology, 15*, 320–5.

Brown, D. D. 1981. Gene expression in eukaryotes. *Science, 211*, 667–74.

Brown, M. S., Kovanen, P. T., & Goldstein, J. L. 1981. Regulation of plasma cholesterol by lipoprotein receptors. *Science, 212*, 628–35.

Buell, S. J., & Coleman, P. D. 1979. Dendritic growth in the aged human brain and failure of growth in senile dementia. *Science, 206*, 854–6.

Bühler, C. 1928. *Kindheit und Jugend*. Leipzig: S. Herzel.

Bullough, V. L. 1981. Age at menarche: A misunderstanding. *Science, 213*, 365–6.

Burgess, R. L., & Huston, T. L. (Eds.). 1979. *Social exchange in developing relationships*. New York: Academic Press.

Cairns, R. B., & Hood, K. E. 1983. Continuity in social development: A comparative perspective on individual difference prediction. In P. B. Baltes & O. G. Brim, Jr. (Eds.), *Life-span development and behavior* (Vol. 5). New York: Academic Press.

Campbell, D. T. 1975. On the conflicts between biological and social evolution and between psychology and moral tradition. *American Psychologist, 30,* 1103–26.

Campenot, R. B. 1981. Regeneration of neurites in long-term cultures of sympathatic neurons deprived of nerve growth factor. *Science, 214,* 579–81.

Capitanio, J. P., & Leger, D. W. 1979. Evolutionary scales lack utility: A reply to Yarczower and Hazlett. *Psychological Bulletin, 86,* 876–9.

Chang, F. L. F., & Greenough, W. T. 1978. Increased dendritic branching in hemispheres opposite eyes exposed to maze training in split-brain rats. *Society for Neuroscience Abstracts, 4,* 469.

Chang, F. L. F., & Greenough, W. T. 1982. Lateralized effects of monocular training on dendritic branching in adult split-brain rats. *Brain Research, 232,* 283–92.

Changeaux, J. P., & Danchin, A. 1977. Biochemical models for the selective stabilization of developing synapses. In G. A. Cattrell & P.N.R. Usherwood (Eds.), *Synapses.* New York: Academic Press.

Chernick, V., & Craig, R. J. 1982. Naloxone reverses neonatal depression caused by fetal asphyxia. *Science, 215,* 1252–3.

Chess, S. & Thomas, A. 1982. Infant bonding: mystique and reality. *American Journal of Orthopsychiatry, 52,* 213–22.

Clarke, A. M. 1982. Developmental discontinuities: An approach to assessing their nature. In L. A. Bond & J. M. Joffee (Eds.), *Facilitating infant and early childhood development.* Hanover, N.H.: University Press of New England.

Clarke, A. M., & Clarke, A. D. B. (Eds.). 1976. *Early experience: Myth and evidence.* New York: Free Press.

Cline, M. J., Strong, H., Mercola, L., Morse, R., Ruprecht, J., Browne, J., & Salser, W. 1980. Gene transfer in intact animals. *Nature, 284,* 422–5.

Cochran, M. M., & Brassard, J. A. 1979. Child development and personal social networks. *Child Development, 50,* 601–16.

Coe, C. L., Chen, J., Lowe, E. L., Davidson, J. M., & Levine, S. 1981. Hormonal and behavioral changes at puberty in the squirrel monkey. *Hormones and Behavior, 15,* 36–53.

Coe, C. L., & Levine, S. 1981. *Psychoendocrine relationships underlying reproductive behavior in the squirrel monkey.* Manuscript, Stanford University.

Cohen, S. N. 1976. Transposable genetic elements and plasmid evolution. *Nature, 263,* 731–38.

Colby, A. 1978. Evolution of a moral developmental theory. *New Directions for Child Development, 2,* 89–104.

Collis, M. G., & Shepherd, J. T. 1980. Antidepressant drug action and presynaptic α-receptors. *Mayo Clinic Proceedings, 55,* 567–72.

Coss, R. G., & Globus, A. 1978. Spine stems on tectal interneurons in jewel fish are shortened by social stimulation. *Science, 200,* 787–90.

Cotman, C. W., & Nieto-Sampedro, M. 1982. Brain function, synapse renewal, and plasticity. *Annual Review of Psychology, 33,* 371–401.

Cotman, C., & Scheff, S. W. 1979. Compensatory synapse growth in aged animals after neuronal death. *Mechanisms of Aging and Development, 9,* 103–17.

Cowan, W. M. 1979. The development of the brain. *Scientific American, 241,* 113–33.

Cragg, B. G. 1975. The density of synapses and neurons in normal, mentally defective and aging human brains. *Brain, 98,* 81–90.

Crockenberg, S. B. 1981. Infant irritability, mother responsiveness, and social support influences on the security of infant–mother attachment. *Child Development, 52,* 857–65.

Curio, E., Ernst, U., & Vieth, W. 1978. Cultural transmission of enemy recognition: One function of mobbing. *Science, 202,* 899–901.

Darwin, C. 1859. *On the origin of species.* London: J. Murray.

Datan, N., & Ginsberg, L. H. (Eds.). 1975. *Life-span developmental psychology: Normative life crises.* New York: Academic Press.

Datan, N., & Reese, H. W. (Eds.). 1977. *Life-span developmental psychology: Dialectical perspectives on experimental psychology.* New York: Academic Press.

de Beer, G. R. 1959. Paedomorphosis. *Proceedings of the XV International Congress of Zoology, 15,* 927–30.

DeVoogd, T., & Nottebohm, F. 1981. Gonadal hormones induce dendritic growth in the adult avian brain. *Science, 214,* 202–4.

Diamond, M. C. 1967. Extensive cortical depth measurements and neuron size increases in the cortex of environmentally enriched rats. *Journal of Comparative Neurology, 131,* 357–64.

Dobzhansky, T., Ayala, F. J., Stebbings, G. L., & Valentine, J. W. 1977. *Evolution.* San Francisco: Freeman.

Doolittle, W. F., & Sapienza, C. 1980. Selfish genes, the phenotype paradigm, and genome evolution. *Nature, 284,* 601–3.

Dornbusch, S. M., Carlsmith, J. M., Gross, R. T., Martin, J. A., Jennings, D., Rosenberg, A., & Duke, P. 1981. Sexual development, age, and dating: A comparison of biological and social influences upon one set of behaviors. *Child Development, 52,* 179–85.

Dunn, J. F. 1980. Individual differences in temperament. In M. Rutter (Ed.), *The scientific foundations of developmental psychiatry.* London: Heinemann Medical Books.

Dyer, F. C., & Gould, J. L. 1981. Honey bee orientation: A backup system for cloudy days. *Science, 214,* 1041–2.

Edwards, D. A. 1970. Postnatal androgenization and adult aggressive behavior in female mice. *Physiology and Behavior, 5,* 1115–19.

Egan, T. M., & North, R. A. 1981. Both μ and δ opiate receptors exist on the same neuron. *Science, 214,* 923–24.

Einhorn, D., Young, J. B., & Landesberg, L. 1982. Hypotensive effect of fasting: Possible involvement of the sympathetic nervous system and endogenous opiates. *Science, 218,* 727–9.

Eisenberg, L. 1972. On the human nature of human nature. *Science, 176,* 123–8.

Elder, G. H., Jr. 1974. *Children of the Great Depression.* Chicago: University of Chicago Press.

Elder, G. H., Jr. 1979. Historical change in life patterns and personality. In P. B. Baltes & O. G. Brim, Jr., (Eds.), *Life-span development and behavior* (Vol. 2). New York: Academic Press.

Elliott, E. J., & Muller, K. J. 1982. Synapses between neurons regenerate accurately after destruction of ensheathing glial cells in the leech. *Science, 215,* 1260–2.

Enna, S. J., Samorajski, T., & Beer, B. (Eds.). 1981. *Aging,* Vol. 17: *Brain neurotransmitters and receptors in aging and age-related disorders.* New York: Raven Press.

Erikson, E. H. 1968. *Identity, youth and crisis.* New York: Norton.

Eveleth, P. B., & Tanner, J. M. 1976. *Worldwide variation in human growth.* Cambridge: Cambridge University Press.

Eysenck, H. J., & Kamin, L. 1981. *Intelligence: The battle for the mind.* New York: Macmillan.

Faden, A. I., Jacobs, T. P., & Holaday, J. W. 1981. Opiate antagonist improves neurological recovery after spinal injury. *Science, 211,* 493–4.

Featherman, D. L. 1981-82. The life-span perspective in social science research. In *The Five Year Outlook in Science and Technology* (Vol. 2). Washington, D.C.: National Science Foundation.

Feener, D. H., Jr. 1981. Competition between ant species: Outcomes controlled by parasitic flies. *Science, 214,* 815–17.

Fiala, B. A., Joyce, J. N., & Greenough, W. T. 1978. Environmental complexity modulates growth of granule cell dendrites in developing but not adult hippocampus of rats. *Experimental Neurology, 59,* 372–83.

Fisher, H. E. 1982a. Of human bonding. *The Sciences, 22,* 18–23, 31.

Fisher, H. E. 1982b. Is it sex? Helen E. Fisher replies. *The Sciences, 22,* 2–3.

Flint, B. M. 1978. *New hope for deprived children.* Toronto: Toronto University Press.

Floeter, M. K., & Greenough, W. T. 1979. Cerebellar plasticity: Modification of Purkinje cell structure by differential rearing in monkeys. *Science, 206,* 227–9.

Fox, L. R., & Morrow, P. A. 1981. Specialization: Species property or local phenomenon? *Science, 211,* 887–93.

Fraiberg, S. 1977. *Every child's birthright: In defense of mothering.* New York: Basic Books.

Franklin, M. B., & Doyle, C. L. 1982. Perspectives on plasticity. *Contemporary Psychology, 27,* 694–5.

French, J. R. P., Jr., Rodgers, W., & Cobb, S. 1974. Adjustment as person-environment fit. In G. V. Coelho, D. A. Hamburg, & J. E. Adams (Eds.), *Coping and adaptation.* New York: Basic Books.

Freeman, R. D., & Bonds, A. B. 1979. Cortical plasticity in monocularly deprived immobilized kittens depends on eye movement. *Science, 206,* 1093–5.

Freud, A. 1969. Adolescence as a developmental disturbance. In G. Caplan & S. Lebovici (Eds.), *Adolescence.* New York: Basic Books.

Futuyma, D. J. 1982. A synthetic history of biology. *Science, 216,* 842–4.

Gambert, S. R., Garthwaite, T. L., Pontzer, C. H., & Hagen, T. C. 1980. Fasting associated with decrease in hypothalamic beta-endorphin. *Science, 210,* 1271–2.

Garn, S. M. 1980. Continuities and change in maturational timing. In O. G. Brim, Jr., & J. Kagan (Eds.), *Constancy and change in human development.* Cambridge: Harvard University Press.

Gash, D., Sladek, J. R., & Sladek, C. D. 1980. Functional development of grafted vasopressin neurons. *Science, 210,* 1367–9.

Geinisman, Y., & Bondareff, W. 1976. Decrease in the number of synapses in the brain: A quantitative electron microscopic analysis of the dentate gyrus in the rat. *Mechanisms of Aging and Development, 5,* 11–23.

Gilbert, J. J. 1980. Developmental polymorphism in the Rotifer *Asplanchna sieboldi. American Scientist, 68,* 636–46.

Gilbert, W. 1981. DNA sequencing and gene structure. *Science, 214,* 1305–12.

Glick, R., & Bondareff, W. 1979. Loss of synapses in the cerebellar cortex of the senescent rat. *Journal of Gerontology, 34,* 818–22.

Globus, A. 1975. Brain morphology as a function of presynaptic morphology and activity. In A. Riesen (Ed.), *The developmental neuropsychology of sensory deprivation.* New York: Academic Press.

Globus, A., Rosenzweig, M. R., Bennett, E. L., & Diamond, M. C. 1973. Effects of differential experience on dendritic spine counts in rat cerebral cortex. *Journal of Comparative and Physiological Psychology, 82,* 175–81.

Globus, A., & Scheibel, A. B. 1967. Synaptic loci on parietal cortical neurons: Termination of corpus callosum fibers. *Science, 156,* 1127–9.

Goddard, H. H. 1912. *The Kallikak family: A study in the heredity of feeble-mindedness.* New York: Macmillan.

Goddard, H. H. 1914. *Feeble-mindedness: Its causes and consequences.* New York: Macmillan.

Goldsmith, H. H., & Campos, J. 1981. Toward a theory of infant temperament. In R. N. Emde & R. Harmon (Eds.), *Attachment and affiliative systems: Neurobiological and psychobiological aspects.* New York: Plenum Press.

Goldstein, A., Lowney, L. I., & Pal, B. K. 1971. Stereospecific and nonspecific interactions of the morphine congener leverphanol in subcellular fractions of mouse brain. *Proceedings of the National Academy of Science, 68,* 1742–7.

Gollin, E. S. 1981. Development and plasticity. In E. S. Gollin (Ed.), *Developmental plasticity: Behavioral and biological aspects of variations in development.* New York: Academic Press.

Goodenow, R. S., McMillan, A., Örn, M., Nicholson, M., Davidson, N., Frelinger, J. A., & Hood, L. 1982. Identification of a BALB/C H-2L^d gene by DNA-mediated gene transfer. *Science, 215,* 677–9.

Gordon, J. W., Scangos, G. A., Plotkin, D. J., Barbosa, J. A., & Ruddle, F. H. In press. Genetic transformation of mouse embryos by microinjection of purified DNA. *Proceedings of the National Academy of Science.*

Gottlieb, G. 1970. Conceptions of prenatal behavior. In L. R. Aronson, E. Tobach, D. S. Lehrman, & J. S. Rosenblatt (Eds.), *Development and evolution of behavior: Essays in memory of T. C. Schneirla.* San Francisco: Freeman.

Gottlieb, G. 1976a. The roles of experience in the development of behavior and the nervous system. In G. Gottlieb (Ed.), *Neural and behavioral specificity: Studies on the development of behavior and the nervous system* (Vol. 3). New York: Academic Press.

Gottlieb, G. 1976b. Conceptions of prenatal development: Behavioral embryology. *Psychological Review. 83*, 215–34.

Gould, S. J. 1976. Grades and clades revisited. In R. B. Masterton, W. Hodos, & H. Jerison (Eds.), *Evolution, brain, and behavior: Persistent problems.* Hillsdale, N.J.: Erlbaum.

Gould, S. J. 1977. *Ontogeny and phylogeny.* Cambridge: Belknap Press of Harvard University Press.

Gould, S. J. 1981. *The mismeasure of man.* New York: Norton.

Gould, S. J., & Lewontin, R. C. 1979. The spandrels of San Marco and the Panglossian paradigm: A critique of the adaptationist programme. In J. Maynard Smith & R. Holliday (Eds.), *The evolution of adaptation by natural selection.* London: Royal Society of London.

Gould, S., & Vrba, E. 1982. Exaptation: A missing term in the science of form. *Paleobiology, 8*, 4–15.

Goulet, L. R., & Baltes, P. B. (Eds.). 1970. *Life-span developmental psychology: Research and theory.* New York: Academic Press.

Graf, L. H., Jr. 1982. Gene transformation. *American Scientist, 70*, 496–505.

Grau, J. W., Hyson, R. L., Maier, S. F., Madden IV, J., & Barchas, J. D. 1981. Long-term stress-induced analgesia and activation of the opiate system. *Science, 213*, 1409–11.

Graziadei, P. P. C., & Monti-Graziadei, G. A. 1978. The olfactory system: A model for the study of neurogenesis and axon regeneration in mammals. In C. W. Cotman (Ed.), *Neuronal plasticity.* New York: Raven.

Graziadei, P. P. C., & Monti-Graziadei, G. A. 1979. Neurogenesis and neuron regeneration in the olfactory system of mammals. I. Morphological aspects of differentiation and structural organization of the olfactory sensory neurons. *Journal of Neurocytology, 8*, 1–17.

Greenough, W. T. 1975. Experimental modification of the developing brain. *American Scientist, 63*, 37–46.

Greenough, W. T. 1978. Development and memory: The synaptic connection. In T. Teyler (Ed.), *Brain and learning.* Stamford, Conn.: Greylock Publishers.

Greenough, W. T., & Green, E. J. 1981. Experience and the changing brain. In J. L. McGaugh, J. G. March, & S. B. Kiesler (Eds.), *Aging: Biology and behavior.* New York: Academic Press.

Greenough, W. T., Juraska, J. M., & Volkmar, F. R. 1979. Maze training effects on dendritic branching in occipital cortex of adult rats. *Behavioral and Neural Biology, 26,* 287–97.

Greenough, W. T., & Volkmar, F. R. 1973. Pattern of dendritic branching in occipital cortex of rats reared in complex environments. *Experimental Neurology, 40*, 491–504.

Grouse, L. D., Schrier, B. K., & Nelson, P. G. 1979. Effect of visual experience on gene expression during the development of stimulus specificity in cat brain. *Experimental neurology, 64*, 354–64.

Grouse, L. D., Schrier, B. K., Bennett, E. L., Rosenzweig, M. R., & Nelson, P. G. Sequence diversity studies of rat brain RNA: Effects of environmental complexity and rat brain RNA diversity. *Journal of Neurochemistry, 30*, 191–203.

Haan, N. 1981. Adolescents and young adults as producers of their development. In R. M. Lerner & N. A. Busch-Rossnagel (Eds.), *Individuals as producers of their development: A life-span perspective.* New York: Academic Press.

Haeckel, E. 1868. *Natürliche Schöpfringsgeschichte*. Berlin: Reimer.

Hall, G. S. 1904. *Adolescence: Its psychology and its relations to physiology, anthropology, sociology, sex, crime, religion, and education* (Vols. 1 and 2). New York: Appleton.

Harley, D. 1982. Models of human evolution. *Science, 217*, 296.

Harrell, R. F., Capp, R. H., Davis, D. R., Peerless, J., & Ravitz, L. R. 1981. Can nutritional supplements help mentally retarded children? An exploratory study. *Proceedings of the National Academy of Science, 78*, 574–8.

Harris, D. B. (Ed.). 1957. *The concept of development*. Minneapolis: University of Minnesota Press.

Harrison, R. V. 1978. Person–environment fit and job stress. In C. L. Cooper & R. Payne (Eds.), *Stress at work*. New York: Wiley.

Hartup, W. W. 1978. Perspectives on child and family interaction: Past, present, and future. In R. M. Lerner & G. B. Spanier (Eds.), *Child influences on marital and family interaction: A life-span perspective*. New York: Academic Press.

Hayes, R. L., Bennett, G. J., Newlon, P. G., & Mayer, D. J. 1978. Behavioral and physiological studies of non-narcotic analgesia in the rat elicited by certain environmental stimuli. *Brain Research, 155*, 69–90.

Hebb, D. O. 1949. *The organization of behavior*. New York: Wiley.

Hebb, D. O., & Williams, K. 1946. A method of rating animal intelligence. *Journal of General Psychology, 34*, 59–65.

Held, R., & Hein, A. V. 1963. Movement-produced stimulation in the development of visually guided behavior. *Journal of Comparative and Physiological Psychology, 56*, 872–6.

Hemmes, R. B., Pack, H. M., Hirsch, J. 1979. Chronic ingestion of L-dopa dramatically reduces body weight of the genetically obese Zucker rat. *Federation Proceedings, 38*, 277.

Hempel, C. G. 1966. *Philosophy of natural science*. Englewood Cliffs, N.J.: Prentice-Hall.

Henderson, L. J. 1913. *The fitness of the environment*. New York: Macmillan.

Herman, B. H., & Panksepp, J. 1980. Ascending endorphin inhibition of distress vocalization. *Science, 211*, 1060–7.

Hill, R., & Mattessich, P. 1979. Family development theory and life-span development. In P. B. Baltes & O. G. Brim, Jr., (Eds.), *Life-span development and behavior* (Vol. 2). New York: Academic Press.

Hirsch, J. 1970. Behavior–genetic analysis and its biosocial consequences. *Seminars in Psychiatry, 2*, 89–105.

Hoffman, H., & Rattner, A. 1973. A reinforcement model of imprinting. *Psychological Review, 80*, 527–44.

Hogan, R., Johnson, J. A., & Emler, N. P. 1978. A socioanalytic theory of moral development. *New Directions for Child Development, 2*, 1–18.

Högstedt, G. 1980. Evolution of clutch size in birds: Adaptive variation in relation to territory quality. *Science, 210*, 1148–50.

Holliday, R., Huschtscha, L. I., & Kirkwood, T. B. L. 1981. Cellular aging: Further evidence for the commitment theory. *Science, 213*, 1505–8.

Holloway, R. L., Jr. 1966. Dendritic branching: Some preliminary results of training and complexity in rat visual cortex. *Brain Research, 2*, 393–6.

Holroyd, K. A., Appel, M. A., & Andrasik, F. In press. A cognitive behavioral approach to psychophysiological disorders. In D. Meichenbaum & M. Jaremko (Eds.), *Stress prevention and management: A cognitive behavioral approach*. New York: Plenum Press.

Homans, G. C. 1974. *Social behavior: Its elementary forms* (rev. ed.). New York: Harcourt Brace Jovanovich.

Hoogland, J. L. 1982. Prairie dogs avoid extreme inbreeding. *Science, 215*, 1639–41.

Hosobuchi, Y., Adams, J. E., & Linchitz, R. 1977. Pain relief by electrical stimulation of the central gray matter in humans and its reversal by naloxone. *Science, 197*, 183–6.

Hosobuchi, Y., Baskin, D. S., & Woo, S. K. 1982. Reversal of induced ischemic neurological defect in gerbils by the opiate antagonist naloxone. *Science*, 215, 69–71.

Howard-Flanders, P. 1981. Inducible repair of DNA. *Scientific American*, 245, 72–80.

Hubbard, R. 1982. The ethics and politics of embryo and gene manipulations. *Abstracts of Papers of the 148th National Meeting of the American Association for the Advancement of Science* (abstract).

Hubel, D. H., Wiesel, T. N., & Levay, S. 1977. Plasticity of ocular dominance columns in monkey striate cortex. *Philosophical Transactions of the Royal Society of London*, Series B, 278, 377–409.

Hughes, J., Smith, T., Kosterlitz, H. W., Fothergill, L. A., Morgan, B. A., & Morris, H. 1975. Identification of two related pentapeptides from the brain with potent opiate agonist activity. *Nature*, 258, 577–9.

Hull, C. L. 1952. *A behavior system*. New Haven: Yale University Press.

Hunt, J. McV. 1961. *Intelligence and experience*. New York: Ronald Press.

Hutchinson, G. E. 1981. Random adaptation and imitation in human evolution. *American Scientist*, 69, 161–5.

Huxley, J. S. 1958. Cultural process and evolution. In A. Roe & G. G. Sampson (Eds.), *Behavior and evolution*. New Haven: Yale University Press.

Immelmann, K., & Suomi, S. 1981. Sensitive phases in development. In K. Immelmann, G. Barlow, L. Petrenovich, & M. Main (Eds.), *Behavioral development*. New York: Cambridge University Press.

Isaac, G. L. 1982. Models of human evolution. *Science*, 217, 295.

Iversen, L. L. 1979. The chemistry of the brain. *Scientific American*, 241, 134–49.

Jackson, P. C., & Diamond, J. 1981. Regenerating axons reclaim sensory targets from collateral nerve sprouts. *Science*, 214, 926–8.

Jacob, F., & Monod, J. 1961. On the regulation of gene activity. *Cold Spring Harbor Symposia on Quantitative Biology*, 26, 193–209.

Jacobson, M. 1969. Development of specific neuronal connections. *Science*, 163, 543–7.

Jenkins, J. J. 1974. Remember that old theory of memory? Well forget it. *American Psychologist*, 29, 785–95.

Jerison, H. J. 1978. *Smart dinosaurs and comparative psychology*. Paper presented at the meeting of the American Psychological Association, Toronto, August.

Johanson, D. C., & Edey, M. A. 1981. *Lucy: The beginnings of humankind*. New York: Simon & Schuster.

Jonakait, G. M., Bohn, M. C., & Black, I. B. 1980. Maternal glucocorticoid hormones influence neurotransmitter phenotypic expression in embryos. *Science*, 210, 551–3.

Jones, W. T. 1965. *The sciences and the humanities: Conflict and reconciliation*. Berkeley: University of California Press.

Juraska, J. M., Greenough, W. T., Elliott, C., Mack, K. J., & Berkowitz, R. 1980. Plasticity in adult rat visual cortex: An examination of several cell populations after differential rearing. *Behavioral and Neural Biology*, 29, 157–67.

Kacerguis, M. A. 1982. Child–mother relations in early adolescence: The roles of pubertal status, timing of menarche, and temperament. Ph.D. dissertation. Pennsylvania State University.

Kagan, J. 1966. Reflection–impulsivity: The generality and dynamics of conceptual tempo. *Journal of Abnormal Psychology*, 71, 17–24.

Kagan, J. 1980. Perspectives on continuity. In O. G. Brim, Jr., & J. Kagan (Eds.), *Constancy and change in human development*. Cambridge: Harvard University Press.

Kagan, J. 1983. The premise of connectivity. In R. M. Lerner (Ed.), *Developmental psychology: Historical and philosophical perspectives*. Hillsdale, N.J.: Erlbaum.

Kagan, J., & Moss, H. 1962. *Birth to maturity*. New York: Wiley.

Kandel, E. R., & Schwartz, J. H. (Eds.). 1981. *Principles of neural science*. New York: Elsevier.

Kaplan, B. 1983. A trio of trials. In R. M. Lerner (Ed.), *Developmental psychology: Historical and philosophical perspectives*. Hillsdale, N.J.: Erlbaum.

Kasamatsu, T., & Pettigrew, J. D. 1979. Preservation of binocularity after monocular deprivation in the striate cortex of kittens treated with 6-hydroxydopamine. *Journal of Comparative Neurology, 185*, 139–62.

Katchadourian, H. 1977. *The biology of adolescence*. San Francisco: Freeman.

Kaufmann, H. 1968. *Introduction to the study of human behavior*. Philadelphia: Saunders.

Kendall, P. C. 1981. Cognitive–behavioral interventions with children. In B. Lahey & A. E. Kazdin (Eds.), *Advances in child clinical psychology* (Vol. 4). New York: Plenum Press.

Kendall, P. C., & Hollon, S. D. 1979. Cognitive–behavioral interventions: Overview and current status. In P. C. Kendall & S. D. Hollon (Eds.), *Cognitive–behavioral interventions: Theory, research, and procedures*. New York: Academic Press.

Kendall, P. C., Lerner, R. M., & Craighead, W. E. In press. Human development and intervention in childhood psychopathology. *Child development*.

Kesner, R. P., & Novak, J. M. 1982. Serial position curve in rats: Role of the dorsal hippocampus. *Science, 218*, 173–5.

Klaus, M., & Kennell, J. 1976. *Maternal–infant bonding*. St. Louis: Mosby.

Kleckner, N. 1977. Translocatable elements in prokaryotes. *Cell, 11*, 11–23.

Kleckner, N. 1981. Transposable elements in prokaryotes. *Annual Review of Genetics, 15*, 341–404.

Kohlberg, L. 1976. Moral stages and moralization: The cognitive-developmental approach. In T. Lickona (Ed.), *Moral development and behavior: Theory, research, and social issues*. New York: Holt, Rinehart and Winston.

Kohn, M. 1977. *Social competence, symptoms and underachievement in childhood: A longitudinal perspective*. New York: Wiley.

Kohn, M. L., & Schooler, C. 1979. The reciprocal effects of the substantive complexity of work and intellectual flexibility: A longitudinal assessment. In M. W. Riley (Ed.), *Aging from birth to death: Interdisciplinary perspectives*. Boulder, Colo.: Westview Press.

Kolata, G. B. 1976. Brain biochemistry: Effects of diet. *Science, 192*, 41–2.

Kolata, G. B. 1978. Behavioral teratology: Birth defects of the mind. *Science, 207*, 732–4.

Kolata, G. 1982. Grafts correct brain damage. *Science, 217*, 342–4.

Korn, S. 1978. *Temperament, vulnerability, and behavior*. Paper presented at the Louisville Temperament Conference, Louisville, Ky., September.

Krech, P., Rosenzweig, M. R., & Bennett, E. L. 1963. Effects of complex environment and blindness on rat brain. *Archives of Neurology, 8*, 403–12.

Krieger, D. T., & Martin, J. B. 1981a. Brain peptides (first of two pairs). *New England Journal of Medicine, 304*, 876–85.

Krieger, D. T., & Martin, J. B. 1981b. Brain peptides (second of two pairs). *New England Journal of Medicine, 304*, 994–51.

Kuhn, D. 1978. Mechanisms of cognitive and social development: One psychology or two? *Human Development, 21*, 92–118.

Kuhn, T. S. 1970. *The structure of scientific revolutions* (2nd ed.). Chicago: University of Chicago Press.

Kulka, R. A. 1979. Interaction as person–environment fit. In L. R. Kahle (Ed.), *New directions for methodology of behavioral science: Methods for studying person-situation interactions* (No. 2). San Francisco: Jossey–Bass.

Kulka, R. A., Klingel, D. M., & Mann, D. W. 1980. School crime and disruption as a function of student-school fit: An empirical assessment. *Journal of Youth and Adolescence, 9*, 353–69.

Kunkel, T. A., & Loeb, L. A. 1981. Fidelity of mammalian DNA polymerases. *Science, 213*, 765–7.

Kunos, G., Farsang, C., & Ramirez-Gonzales, M. D. 1981. Beta-endorphin: Possible involvement in the antihypertensive effect of central alpha-receptor activation. *Science, 211*, 82–4.

Lamb, M. E. (Ed.). 1981. *The role of the father in child development* (2nd ed.). New York: Wiley.

Landfield, P. W., Baskin, R. K., & Pitler, T. A. 1981. Brain aging correlates: Retardation by hormonal-pharmacological treatments. *Science, 214*, 581–4.

Lapin, B. A., Krilova, R. I., Cherkovich, G. M., & Asanov, N. S. 1979. Observations from Sukhumi. In D. M. Bowden (Ed.), *Aging in nonhuman primates*. New York: Van Nostrand Reinhold.

Lauder, J. M., & Krebs, H. 1978. Serotonin as a differentiation signal in early neurogenesis. *Developmental Neuroscience, 1*, 15–30.

Lazar, I., Darlington, R., Murray, H., Royce, J., & Snipper, A. 1982. Lasting effects of early education: A report from the consortium for longitudinal studies. *Monographs of the Society for Research in Child Development, 47* (Serial No. 195, Nos. 2–3).

Legros, J. J., Gilot, P., Seron, X., Claessens, J., Adam, A., Moeglen, J. M., Audibert, A., & Berchier, P. 1978. Influence of vasopressin on learning and memory. *Lancet, 1*, 41–2.

Lehrman, D. S. 1953. A critique of Konrad Lorenz's theory of instinctive behavior. *Quarterly Review of Biology, 28*, 337–63.

Lehrman, D. S. 1970. Semantic and conceptual issues in the nature-nurture problem. In L. R. Aronson, E. Tobach, D. S. Lehrman, & J. S. Rosenblatt (Eds.), *Development and evolution of behavior: Essays in memory of T. C. Schneirla*. San Francisco: Freeman.

Lerner, J. V. 1983. The role of temperament in psychosocial adaptation in early adolescents: A test of a "goodness of fit" model. *Journal of Genetic Psychology, 143*, 149–57.

Lerner, J. V., & Lerner, R. M. 1983. Temperament and adaptation across life: Theoretical and empirical issues. In P. B. Baltes & O. G. Brim, Jr. (Eds.), *Life-span development and behavior* (Vol. 5). New York: Academic Press.

Lerner, J. V., Lerner, R. M., & Zabski, S. In press. Temperament and elementary school children's actual and rated academic performance: A test of a "goodness of fit" model. *Journal of Child Psychology and Psychiatry*.

Lerner, R. M. 1976. *Concepts and theories of human development*. Reading, Mass.: Addison-Wesley.

Lerner, R. M. 1978. Nature, nurture, and dynamic interactionism. *Human Development, 21*, 1–20.

Lerner, R. M. 1979. A dynamic interactional concept of individual and social relationship development. In R. L. Burgess & T. L. Huston (Eds.), *Social exchange in developing relationships*. New York: Academic Press.

Lerner, R. M. 1980. Concepts of epigenesis: Descriptive and explanatory issues. A critique of Kitchner's comments. *Human Development, 23*, 63–72.

Lerner, R. M. 1982. Children and adolescents as producers of their own development. *Developmental Review, 2*, 342–70.

Lerner, R. M. In press. Individual and context in developmental psychology: Conceptual and empirical issues. In J. R. Nesselroade & A. von Eye (Eds.), *Individual development and social change: Explanatory analysis*. New York: Academic Press.

Lerner, R. M., & Busch-Rossnagel, N. 1981. Individuals as producers of their development: Conceptual and empirical bases. In R. M. Lerner & N. A. Busch-Rossnagel (Eds.), *Individuals as producers of their development: A life-span perspective*. New York: Academic Press.

Lerner, R. M., & Hultsch, D. F. 1983. *Human development: A life-span perspective*. New York: McGraw-Hill.

Lerner, R. M., Hultsch, D. F., & Dixon, R. A. 1983. Contextualism and the character of developmental psychology in the 1970s. *Annals of the New York Academy of Sciences, 412*, 101–28.

Lerner, R. M., & Lerner, J. V. 1984. *Children in their contexts: A goodness of fit model*. Paper prepared for forthcoming Social Science Research Council-Sponsored volume on "Life-Span Approaches to Parental and Offspring Development."

Lerner, R. M., Palermo, M., Spiro, A., III, & Nesselroade, J. R. 1982. Assessing the dimensions of temperamental individuality across the life-span: The Dimensions of Temperament Survey (DOTS). *Child Development, 53*, 149–59.

Lerner, R. M., & Ryff, C. D. 1978. Implementation of the life-span view of human development: The sample case of attachment. In P. B. Baltes (Ed.), *Life-span development and behavior* (Vol. 1). New York: Academic Press.

Lerner, R. M., Skinner, E. A., & Sorrell, G. T. 1980. Methodological implications of contextual/ dialectic theories of development. *Human Development, 23*, 225–35.

Lerner, R. M., & Spanier, G. B. (Eds.). 1978. *Child influences on marital and family interaction: A life-span perspective.* New York: Academic Press.

Levin, P., Janda, J. K., Jospeh, J. A., Ingram, D. K., & Roth, G. S. 1981. Dietary restriction retards the age-associated loss of rat striatal dopaminergic receptors. *Science, 214*, 561–2.

Levine, J. D., Gordon, N. C., & Fields, H. L. 1978. The mechanism of placebo analgesia. *Lancet*, September 23, 654–7.

LeVine, R. A. 1977. Child rearing as cultural adaptation. In P. H. Leiderman, S. R. Tulkin, & A. Rosenfeld (Eds.). *Culture and infancy: Variations in the human experience.* New York: Academic Press.

Levinger, G., & Snoek, J. D. 1972. *Attraction in relationship: A new look at interpersonal attraction.* New York: General Learning Press.

Lewin, R. 1981a. Jumping genes help trace inherited diseases. *Science, 211*, 690–2.

Lewin, R. 1981b. Do jumping genes make evolutionary leaps? *Science, 213*, 634–6.

Lewin, R. 1982a. Biology is not postage stamp collecting. *Science, 216*, 718–20.

Lewin, R. 1982b. How did humans evolve big brains? *Science, 216*, 840–1.

Lewin, R. 1982c. Darwin died at a most propitious time. *Science, 217*, 717–18.

Lewin, R. 1982d. Molecules come to Darwin's aid. *Science, 216*, 1091–2.

Lewin, R. 1982e. Can genes jump between eukaryotic species? *Science, 217*, 42–3.

Lewis, M., & Brooks-Gunn, J. 1979. *Social cognition and the acquisition of self.* New York: Plenum Press.

Lewis, M., & Rosenblum, L. A. (Eds.). 1974. *The effect of the infant on its caregiver.* New York: Wiley.

Lewontin, R. C. 1981. On constraints and adaptation. *Behavioral and Brain Sciences, 4*, 244–5.

Lewontin, R. C., & Levins, R. 1978. Evolution. *Encyclopedia*, Vol. 5, *Divino-Fame*. Torino, Italy: Einaudi.

Liben, L. S., Patterson, A. H., & Newcombe, N. (Eds.). 1981. *Spatial representation and behavior across the life span.* New York: Academic Press.

Lichtman, J. W. 1977. The reorganization of synaptic connexions in the rat submandibular ganglion during postnatal development. *Journal of Physiology* (London), *273*, 155–77.

Liebeskind, J. C., Guilband, G., Besson, J. M., & Oliveras, J. L. 1973. Analgesia from electrical stimulation of the periaqueductal gray matter in the cat: Behavioral observations and inhibitory effects on spinal cord interneurons. *Brain Research, 50*, 441–4.

Liebeskind, J. C., Mayer, D. J., & Akil, H. 1974. Central mechanisms of pain inhibition: Studies from focal brain stimulation. In J. J. Bonica (Ed.), *Advances in neurology*, Vol. 4, *Pain*. New York: Raven Press.

Lorenz, K. 1940. Durch domestikation verusachte störungen arteigenen verhaltens. *Zeitschrift für Angewandte Psychologie und Charakterkunde, 59*, 2–81.

Lorenz, K. 1965. *Evolution and modification of behavior.* Chicago: University of Chicago Press.

Lorenz, K. 1966. *On aggression.* New York: Harcourt, Brace & World.

Lorenz, K. 1971. *Studies in human and animal behavior* (Vol. 2). Cambridge: Harvard University Press.

Lovejoy, C. O. 1981. The origin of man. *Science, 211*, 341–50.

Lozovsky, D., Saller, C. F., & Kopin, I. J. 1981. Dopamine receptor binding is increased in diabetic rats. *Science, 214*, 1031–3.

Lynch, G., & Gall, C. 1979. Organization and reorganization in the central nervous system: Evolving concepts of brain plasticity. In F. T. Falkner & J. M. Tanner (Eds.), *Human growth*, Vol. 3: *Neurobiology and nutrition*. New York: Plenum Press.

Lynch, G., & Gerling, S. 1981. Aging and brain plasticity. In J. L. McGaugh, J. G. March, & S. B. Kiesler (Eds.), *Aging: Biology and behavior*: New York: Academic Press.

Mac Donald, K. 1982. *Models of early experience and sensitive periods: Theory and data*. Manuscript, University of Illinois at Urbana–Champaign.

Madden, J., IV, Akil, H., Patrick, R. L., & Barchas, J. D. 1977. Stress induced parallel changes in central opioid levels and pain responsiveness in the rat. *Nature, 266*, 358–60.

Magnusson, D. (Ed.). 1981. *Toward a psychology of situations: An interactional perspective*. Hillsdale, N.J.: Erlbaum.

Magnusson, D., & Allen, V. L. (Eds.). 1983. *Human development: An interactional perspective*. New York: Academic Press.

Maier, N.R.F., & Schneirla, T. C. 1935. *Principles of animal behavior*. New York: McGraw-Hill.

Mandenoff, A., Fumeron, F., Apfelbaum, M., & Margules, D. L. 1982. Endogenous opiates and energy balance. *Science, 215*, 1536–7.

Martinez, J. L., Jr., Jensen, R. A., Messing, R. B., Rigter, H., & McGaugh, J. L. (Eds.). 1981. *Endogenous peptides and learning and memory processes*. New York: Academic Press.

Martinez, J. L., & Rigter, H. 1980. Endorphins after acquisition and consolidation of an inhibitory avoidance response in rats. *Neuroscience Letter, 19*, 197–201.

Marx, J. L. 1980. Gene transfer moves ahead. *Science, 210*, 1334–6.

Marx, J. L. 1981a. Gene control puzzle begins to yield. *Science, 212*, 653–5.

Marx, J. L. 1981b. More progress on gene transfer. *Science, 213*, 996–7.

Marx, J. L. 1981c. Globin gene transferred. *Science, 213*, 1488.

Marx, J. L. 1981d. Brain opiates in mental illness. *Science, 214*, 1013–15.

Marx, J. L. 1982a. Tracking genes in developing mice. *Science, 215*, 44–7.

Marx, J. L. 1982b. Transplants as guides to brain development. *Science, 217*, 340–2.

Marx, J. L. 1982c. How the brain controls birdsong. *Science, 217*, 1125–6.

Masters, R. D. 1978. Jean-Jacques is alive and well: Rousseau and contemporary sociobiology. *Daedalus, 107*, 93–105.

Mauk, M. D., Warren, J. T., & Thompson, R. F. 1982. Selective, naloxone-reversible morphine depression of learned behavioral and hippocampal responses. *Science, 216*, 434–6.

Mayer, D. J., Wolfle, T. L., Akil, H., Carder, B., & Liebeskind, J. C. 1971. Analgesia from electrical stimulation in the brainstem of the rat. *Science, 174*, 1351–4.

Maynard-Smith, J. 1982. Overview – unsolved evolutionary problems. In G. A. Dover & R. B. Flavell (Eds.), *Genome evolution*. New York: Academic Press.

Mayr, E. 1982. *The growth of biological thought*. Cambridge: Harvard University Press.

McClearn, G. E. 1970. Genetic influences on behavior and development. In P. Mussen (Ed.), *Carmichael's manual of child psychology* (Vol. 1). New York: Wiley.

McClearn, G. E. 1981. Evolution and genetic variability. In E. S. Gollin (Ed.), *Developmental plasticity: Behavioral and biological aspects of variations in development*. New York: Academic Press.

McClintock, M. K. 1971. Menstrual synchrony and suppression. *Nature, 229*, 224–5.

McClintock, J. M. 1981. Social control of the ovarian cycle and the function of estrous synchrony. *American Zoologist, 21*, 243–56.

McKay, H., Sinisterra, L., McKay, A., Gomez, H., & Lloreda, P. 1978. Improving cognitive ability in chronically deprived children. *Science, 200*, 270–8.

McKnight, S., & Kinsbury, R. 1982. Transcriptional control signals of a eukaryotic protein-coding gene. *Science, 217*, 316–24.

McKusick, V. A. 1981. The anatomy of the human genome. *Hospital Practice*, 82–100.

Meacham, J. A. 1976. Continuing the dialogue: Dialectics and remembering. *Human Development, 19*, 304–9.

Meacham, J. A. 1977. A transactional model of remembering. In N. Datan & H. W. Reese (Eds.), *Life-span developmental psychology: Dialectical perspective on experimental research*. New York: Academic Press.

Mead, G. H. 1934. *Mind, self, and society*. Chicago: University of Chicago Press.

Meisel, R. L., & Ward, I. L. 1981. Fetal female rats are masculinized by male littermates located caudally in the uterus. *Science, 213*, 239–42.

Mercola, K. E., & Cline, M. J. 1980. Techniques for inserting new genetic information. *New England Journal of Medicine, 303*, 1297–300.

Mercola, K. E., Stang, H. D., Browne, J., Salser, W., & Cline, M. J. 1980. Insertion of a new gene of viral origin into bone marrow cells of mice. *Science, 208*, 1033–5.

Miczek, K. A., Thompson, M. L., & Shuster, L. 1982. Opioid-like analgesia in defeated mice. *Science, 215*, 1520–2.

Mischel, W. 1977. On the future of personality measurement. *American Psychologist, 32*, 246–54.

Moore, K. W., Sher, B. T., Sun, Y. H., Eakle, K. A., & Hood, L. 1982. DNA sequence of a gene encoding a BALB/c mouse L^d transplantation antigen. *Science, 215*, 679-82.

Morgan, B. L. G., & Winick, M. 1980. Effects of environmental stimulation on brain N-acetyl-neuraminic acid content and behavior. *Journal of Nutrition, 110*, 425–32.

Morley, J. E., & Levine, A. S. 1981. Endogenous opiates and stress-induced eating. *Science, 214*, 1150–1.

Murphy, M. R., MacLean, P. D., & Hamilton, S. C. 1981. Species-typical behavior of hamsters deprived from birth of the neocortex. *Science, 213*, 459–61.

Nagel, E. 1957. Determinism and development. In D. B. Harris (Ed.), *The concept of development*. Minneapolis: University of Minnesota Press.

Nerem, R. M., Levesque, M. J., & Cornhill, J. F. 1980. Social environment as a factor in diet-induced atherosclerosis. *Science, 208*, 1475–6.

Nesselroade, J. R., & Baltes, P. B. 1974. Adolescent personality development and historical change, 1970–1972. *Monographs of the Society for Research in Child Development, 39* (1, Serial No. 154).

Nesselroade, J. R., & Reese, H. W. (Eds.). 1973. *Life-span developmental psychology: Methodological issues*. New York: Academic Press.

Nieto-Sampedro, M., Lewis, E. R., Cotman, C. W., Manthorpe, M., Skaper, S. D., Barbin, G., Longo, F. M., & Varon, S. 1982. Brain injury causes a time-dependent increase in neurotrophic activity at the lesion site. *Science, 217*, 860–1.

Nisbet, R. 1980. *History of the idea of progress*. New York: Basic Books.

Nottebohm, F. 1981. A brain for all seasons: Cyclical anatomical changes in song control nuclei of the canary brain. *Science, 214*, 1368–70.

O'Brien, S. J., & Nash, W. G. 1982. Genetic mapping in mammals: Chromosome map of domestic cat. *Science, 216*, 257–65.

Oliveros, J. C., Jandali, M. K., Timsit-Berthier, M., Remey, R., Benghezal, A., Audibert, A., & Moeglen, J. M. 1978. Vasopressin in amnesia. *Lancet, 1*, 42.

Orgel, L. E., & Crick, F. H. C. 1980. Selfish DNA: The ultimate parasite. *Nature, 284*, 604–7.

Overton, W. F. 1978. Klaus Riegel: Theoretical contribution to concepts of stability and change. *Human Development, 21*, 360–3.

Overton, W. F. In press. World views and their influence on scientific research: Kuhn, Lakatos, Lauden. In H. W. Reese (Ed.), *Advances in child development and behavior*. New York: Academic Press.

Overton, W. F., & Reese, H. W. 1973. Models of development: Methodological implications. In J. R. Nesselroade & H. W. Reese (Eds.), *Life-span developmental psychology: Methodological issues*. New York: Academic Press.

Overton, W. & Reese, H. 1981. Conceptual prerequisites for an understanding of stability-change and continuity-discontinuity. *The International Journal of Behavioral Development, 4*, 99–123.

Palermo, M. E. 1982. *Child temperament and contextual demands: A test of the goodness-of-fit model*. Ph.D. dissertation, Pennsylvania State University.

Panksepp, J., Herman, B., Conner, R., Bishop, P., & Scott, J. P. 1978. The biology of social attachments: Opiates alleviate separation distress. *Biological Psychiatry, 13*, 607–18.

Parke, R. D. 1977. Socialization into child abuse: A social interactional perspective. In J. L. Tapp & P. J. Levine (Eds.), *Law, justice, and the individual in society: Psychological and legal issues*. New York: Holt, Rinehart & Winston.

Parke, R. D. 1978. Parent–infant interaction: Progress, paradigms, and problems. In G. P. Sackett (Ed.), *Observing behavior*, Vol. 1: *Theory and applications in mental retardation*. Baltimore: University Park Press.

Parke, R. D. 1979. Perspectives on father–infant interaction. In J. Osofsky (Ed.), *Handbook of infant development*. New York: Wiley.

Parke, R. D. 1981a. *Fathers*. Cambridge: Harvard University Press.

Parke, R. D. 1981b. Father–infant interaction in a family perspective. In P. Berman (Ed.), *Women: A developmental perspective*. Washington, D.C.: U.S. Government Printing Office.

Parke, R. D., Grossman, K., & Tinsley, B. R. 1981. Father–mother–infant interaction in the new-born period: A German-American comparison. In T. Field (Ed.), *Culture and early interactions*. Hillsdale, N.J.: Erlbaum.

Parke, R. D., Hymel, S., Power, T. G., & Tinsley, B. R. 1980. Fathers and risk: A hospital based model of intervention. In D. B. Sawin, R. C. Hawkins, L. O. Walker, & J. H. Penticuff (Eds.), *Exceptional infant*, Vol. 4: *Psychosocial risks in infant–environment transactions*. New York: Brunner/Mazel.

Parke, R. D., Power, T. G., & Gottman, J. M. 1979. Conceptualizing and quantifying influence patterns in the family triad. In M. E. Lamb, S. J. Suomi, & G. R. Stephenson (Eds.), *Social interaction analysis: Methodological issues*. Madison: University of Wisconsin Press.

Parke, R. D., & Tinsley, B. R. 1981. The father's role in infancy: Determinants of involvement in care giving and play. In M. E. Lamb (Ed.), *The role of the father in child development* (2nd. ed.). New York: Wiley.

Parke, R. D., & Tinsley, B. R. 1982. The early environment of the at-risk infant: Expanding the social context. In D. Bricker (Ed.), *Intervention with at-risk and handicapped infants: From research to application*. Baltimore: University Park Press.

Pedersen, F. A. 1981. Father influences viewed in a family context. In M. E. Lamb (Ed.). *The role of the father in child development* (2nd. ed.). New York: Wiley.

Pepper, S. C. 1942. *World hypotheses: A study in evidence*. Berkeley: University of California Press.

Perlow, M. J., Freed, W. J., Hoffer, B. J., Seiger, A., Olson, L., & Wyatt, R. J. 1979. Brain grafts reduce motor abnormalities produced by destruction of nigrostriatal dopamine system. *Science, 204*, 643–6.

Pert, C. B., & Snyder, S. H. 1973. Opiate receptor: Demonstration in nervous tissue. *Science, 179*, 1011–14.

Peters, J. M., Preston-Martin, S., & Yu, M. C. 1981. Brain tumors in children and occupational exposure of parents. *Science, 213*, 235–7.

Petersen, A. C., & Taylor, B. 1980. The biological approach to adolescence. In J. Adelson (Ed.), *Handbook of adolescent psychology*. New York: Wiley.

Petrinovich, L. 1979. Probabilistic functionalism: A conception of research method. *American Psychologist, 34*, 373–90.

Piaget, J. 1961. *Les mecanismes perceptifs*. Paris: Presses Universitaires de France.

Piaget, J., & Inhelder, B. 1956. *The child's conception of space*. London: Routledge.

Plomin, R., & Deitrich, R. A. 1982. Neuropharmacogenetics and behavior genetics. *Behavior Genetics, 12*, 111–21.

Prigogine, I. 1978. Time, structure, and fluctuation. *Science, 201*, 777–85.

Prigogine, I. 1980. *From being to becoming*. San Francisco: Freeman.

Prokopy, R. J., Averill, A. L., Cooley, S. S., & Roitberg, C. A. 1982. Associative learning in egglaying site selection by apple maggot flies. *Science, 218*, 76–7.

Ptashne, M., Johnson, D., & Pabo, C. O. 1982. A genetic switch in a bacterial virus. *Scientific American, 247*, 128–40.

Purves, D., & Lichtman, J. W. 1980. Elimination of synapses in the developing nervous system. *Science, 210*, 153–7.

Ramey, C. T. 1982. Commentary to Lazar et al., "Lasting effects of early education: A report from the consortium for longitudinal studies." *Monographs of the Society for Research in Child Development, 47* (Serial No. 195, Nos. 2–3).

Reddy, E. P., Smith, M. J., & Aaronson, S. A. 1981. Complete nucleotide sequence and organization of the Maloney murine sarcoma virus genome. *Science, 214*, 445–50.

Reese, H. W., & Overton, W. F. 1970. Models of development and theories of development. In L. R. Goulet & P. B. Baltes (Eds.), *Life-span developmental psychology: Research and theory*. New York: Academic Press.

Riegel, K. F. 1975. Toward a dialectical theory of development. *Human Development, 18*, 50–64.

Riegel, K. F. 1976. The dialectics of human development. *American Psychologist, 31*, 689–700.

Riley, M. W. 1978. Aging, social change, and the power of ideas. *Daedalus*, Fall, 39–52.

Riley, M. W. 1979a. Introduction: Life-course perspectives. In M. W. Riley (Ed.), *Aging from birth to death*. Washington, D.C.: American Association for the Advancement of Science.

Riley, M. W. 1979b. Aging, social change, and social policy. In M. W. Riley (Ed.), *Aging from birth to death*. Washington, D.C.: American Association for the Advancement of Science.

Rosenzweig, M. R., & Bennett, E. L. 1977. Effects of environmental enrichment or impoverishment on learning and on brain values in rodents. In A. Oliveiro (Ed.), *Genetics, environment, and intelligence*. Amsterdam: North Holland Biomedical.

Rosenzweig, M. R., & Bennett, E. L. 1978. Experiential influences on brain anatomy and brain chemistry in rodents. In G. Gottlieb (Ed.), *Influences: Studies on the development of behavior and the nervous system*. New York: Academic Press.

Rosenzweig, M. R., Bennett, E. L., & Diamond, M. C. 1972a. Brain changes in response to experience. *Scientific American, 226*, 22–29.

Rosenzweig, M. R., Bennett, E. L., & Diamond, M. C. 1972b. Chemical and anatomical plasticity of brain: Replications and extensions. In J. Gaito (Ed.), *Macromolecules and behavior* (2nd. ed.). New York: Appleton-Century-Crofts.

Rothman-Denes, L. 1982. Transposons. *Science. 215*, 52–53.

Rothshenker, S. 1979. Synapse formation in intact innervated cutaneous-pectoris muscles of the frog following denervation of the opposite muscle. *Journal of Physiology* (London), *292*, 535–47.

Rubin, G. M., & Spradling, A. C. 1982. Genetic transformation of *Drosophila* with transposable element vectors. *Science, 218*, 348–53.

Ruttledge, L. T. 1976. Synaptogenesis: Effects of synaptic use. In M. R. Rosenzweig & E. L. Bennett (Eds.), *Neural mechanisms of learning and memory*. Cambridge: MIT Press.

Ruttledge, L. T., Wright, C., & Duncan, J. 1974. Morphological changes in pyramidal cells of mammalian neocortex associated with increased use. *Experimental Neurology, 44*, 209–28.

Ryder, N. 1965. The cohort as a concept in the study of social change. *American Sociological Review, 30*, 843–61.

Sameroff, A. L. 1975. Transactional models in early social relations. *Human Development, 18*, 65–79.

Sanger, F. 1981. Determination of nucleotide sequences in DNA. *Science, 214*, 1205–10.

Sarason, S. B. 1973. Jewishness, blackishness, and the nature–nurture controversy. *American Psychologist, 28*, 962–71.

Sarbin, T. R. 1977. Contextualism: A world view for modern psychology. In J. K. Cole (Ed.), *Nebraska symposium on motivation, 1976*. Lincoln: University of Nebraska Press.

Scarr, S. 1982. Development is internally guided, not determined. *Contemporary Psychology, 27*, 852–3.

Scarr, S., & McCartney, K. 1983. How people make their own environments: A theory of genotype → environment effects. *Child Development, 54*, 424–35.

Schaie, K. W. 1965. A general model for the study of developmental problems. *Psychological Bulletin, 64*, 92–107.

Schaie, K. W., Anderson, V. E., McClearn, G. E., & Money, J. (Eds). 1975. *Developmental human behavior genetics*. Lexington, Mass.: Heath.

Schaie, K. W., Labouvie, G. V., & Buech, B. V. 1973. Generational and cohort-specific differences in adult cognitive functioning: A fourteen-year study of independent samples. *Developmental Psychology, 9*, 151–66.

Scheff, S. W., Bernardo, L. S., & Cotman, C. W. 1978. Decrease in adrenergic axon sprouting in the senescent rat. *Science, 202*, 775–8.

Schneirla, T. C. 1956. Interrelationships of the innate and the acquired in instinctive behavior. In *L'Instinct dans le comportement des animaux et de l'homme*. Paris: Masson.

Schneirla, T. C. 1957. The concept of development in comparative psychology. In D. B. Harris (Ed.), *The concept of development*. Minneapolis: University of Minnesota Press.

Schneirla, T. C. 1959. An evolutionary and developmental theory of biphasic processes underlying approach and withdrawal. In M. R. Jones (Ed.), *Nebraska symposium on motivation*. Lincoln: University of Nebraska Press.

Schneirla, T. C. 1966. Instinct and aggression. *Natural History, 75*, 16ff.

Schneirla, T. C. 1972. Levels in the psychological capacities of animals. In L. R. Aronson, E. Tobach, J. S. Rosenblatt, & D. S. Lehrman (Eds.), *Selected writings of T. C. Schneirla*. San Francisco: Freeman.

Schopf, T. J. M. 1982. Evolution from the molecular viewpoint. *Science, 217*, 438–40.

Scriver, C. R., & Clow, C. L. 1980a. Phenylketonuria: Epitome of human biochemical genetics (first of two parts). *New England Journal of Medicine, 303*, 1336–42.

Scriver, C. R., & Clow, C. L. 1980b. Phenylketonuria: Epitome of human biochemical genetics (second of two parts). *New England Journal of Medicine, 303*, 1394–1400.

Selkoe, D. J., Ihara, Y., & Salazar, F. J. 1982. Alzheimer's disease: Insolubility of partially purified paired helical filaments in sodium dodecyl sulfate and urea. *Science, 215*, 1243–5.

Sengelaub, D. R., & Finlay, B. L. 1981. Early removal of one eye reduces normally occurring cell death in the remaining eye. *Science, 213*, 573–4.

Sheldon, W. H. 1940. *The varieties of human physique*. New York: Harper.

Sheldon, W. H. 1942. *The varieties of temperament*. New York: Harper.

Sherrington, C. S. 1951. *Man on his nature*. New York: Cambridge University Press.

Sigman, M. 1982. Plasticity in development: Implications for intervention. In L. A. Bond & J. M. Joffe (Eds.), *Facilitating infant and early childhood development*. Hanover, N.H.: University Press of New England.

Simon, E. J., Hiller, J. M., & Edelman, I. 1973. Stereospecific binding of the potent narcotic analgesia (^{3}H)etorphine to rat-brain homogenate. *Proceedings of the National Academy of Science, 70*, 1947–9.

Sklar, L. S., & Anisman, H. 1979. Stress and coping factors influence tumor growth. *Science, 205*, 513–35.

Snow, C. P. 1959. *The two cultures and the scientific revolution.* New York: Cambridge University Press.

Snyder, M. 1981. On the influence of individuals on situations. In N. Cantor & J. F. Kihlstrom (Eds.), *Cognition, social interaction, and personality.* Hillsdale, N.J.: Erlbaum.

Sorell, G. T., & Nowak, C. A. 1981. The role of physical attractiveness as a contributor to individual development. In R. M. Lerner & N. A. Busch-Rossnagel (Eds.), *Individuals as producers of their development: A life-span perspective.* New York: Academic Press.

Spanier, G. B. 1976. Measuring dyadic adjustment: New scales for assessing the quality of marriage and similar dyads. *Journal of Marriage and the Family, 38,* 15–28.

Spanier, G. B., Lerner, R. M., & Aquilino, W. 1978. Future perspectives on child-family inter-actions. In R. M. Lerner & G. B. Spanier (Eds.), *Child influences on marital and family interaction: A life span perspective.* New York: Academic Press.

Sperry, R. W. 1965. Mind, brain, and humanist values. In J. R. Platt (Ed.), *New views of the nature of man.* Chicago: University of Chicago Press.

Sperry, R. W. 1981. Changing priorities. *Annual Review of Neuroscience, 4,* 1–15.

Sperry, R. W. 1982a. Some effects of disconnecting the cerebral hemispheres. *Science, 217,* 1223–6.

Sperry, R. W. 1982b. *Science and moral priority: Merging mind, brain, and human values.* New York: Columbia University Press.

Spinelli, D. N., & Jensen, F. E. 1979. Plasticity: The mirror of experience. *Science, 203,* 75–8.

Sroufe, L. A. 1979. The coherence of individual development. *American Psychologist, 34,* 834–41.

Sroufe, L. A., & Waters, E. 1977. Attachment as an organizational construct. *Child Development, 48,* 1184–99.

Stacey, P. B., & Bock, C. E. 1978. Social plasticity in the acorn woodpecker. *Science, 202,* 1298–300.

Stefano, G. B., Hall, B., Markman, M. H., & Dvorkin, B. 1981. Opioid inhibition of dopamine release from nervous tissue of *Mytilus edulis and Octopus bimaculatus. Science, 213,* 928–30.

Steinberg, L. D., & Hill, J. P. 1978. Patterns of family interaction as a function of age, the onset of puberty, and formal thinking. *Developmental Psychology, 14,* 683–4.

Stern, C. 1973. *Principles of human genetics* (3rd ed.). San Francisco: Freeman.

Streissguth, A. P., Landesman-Dwyer, S., Martin, J. C., & Smith, D. W. 1980. Teratogenic effects of alcohol in humans and laboratory animals. *Science, 209,* 353–61.

Struble, R. G., Cork, L. C., Whitehouse, P. J., & Price, D. L. 1982. Cholinergic innervation in neuritic plaques. *Science, 216,* 413–14.

Super, C. M., & Harkness, S. 1981. Figure, ground and gestalt: The cultural context of the active individual. In R. M. Lerner & N. A. Busch-Rossnagel (Eds.), *Individuals as producers of their development: A life-span perspective.* New York: Academic Press.

Swartz, D. 1982. Is it sex? *The Sciences, 22,* 2.

Terenius, L. 1973. Characteristics of the "receptor" for narcotic analgesics in synaptic plasma membrane fraction from rat brain. *Acta Pharmacological Toxicology, 33,* 377–84.

Terman, L. M. 1916. *The measurement of intelligence.* Boston: Houghton Mifflin.

Thibaut, J. W., & Kelly, H. H. 1961. *The social psychology of groups.* New York: Wiley.

Thomas, A., & Chess, S. 1970. Behavioral individuality in childhood. In L. R. Aronson, E. Tobach, D. S. Lehrman, & J. S. Rosenblatt (Eds.), *Development and evolution of behavior.* San Francisco: Freeman.

Thomas, A., & Chess, S. 1976. Evolution of behavior disorders into adolescence. *American Journal of Psychiatry, 133,* 539–42.

Thomas, A., & Chess, S. 1977. *Temperament and development.* New York: Brunner/Mazel.

Thomas, A., & Chess, S. 1980. *The dynamics of psychological development.* New York: Brunner/Mazel.

Thomas, A., & Chess, S. 1981. The role of temperament in the contributions of individuals to their development. In R. M. Lerner & N. A. Busch-Rossnagel (Eds.), *Individuals as producers of their development: A life-span perspective.* New York: Academic Press.

Thomas, A., Chess, S., & Birch, H. 1968. *Temperament and behavior disorders in children.* New York: New York University Press.

Thomas, A., Chess, S., Birch, H., Hertzig, M., & Korn, S. 1963. *Behavioral individuality in early childhood.* New York: New York University Press.

Thomas, A., Chess, S., Sillan, J., & Mendez, O. 1974. Cross-cultural study of behavior in children with special vulnerabilities to stress. In D. F. Ricks, A. Thomas, & M. Roff (Eds.), *Life history research in psychopathology.* Minneapolis: University of Minnesota Press.

Thompson, R. F. 1981. *The brain.* Manuscript, Stanford University.

Tobach, E. 1978. The methodology of sociobiology from the viewpoint of a comparative psychologist. In A. L. Caplan (Ed.), *The sociobiology debate.* New York: Harper & Row.

Tobach, E., & Schneirla, T. C. 1968. The biopsychology of social behavior of animals. In R. E. Cooke & S. Levin (Eds.), *Biologic basis of pediatric practice.* New York: McGraw-Hill.

Toulmin, S. 1981. Epistemology and developmental psychology. In E. S. Gollin (Ed.), *Developmental plasticity: Behavioral and biological aspects of variations in development.* New York: Academic Press.

Townes-Anderson, E., & Raviola, G. 1976. Giant nerve fibers in the ciliary muscle and iris sphincter of *Macaca mulatta. Cell Tissue Research, 169,* 33–40.

Townes-Anderson, E., & Raviola, G. 1977. Degeneration and regeneration of nerve terminals in the ciliary muscle of primates. *Anatomical Records, 187,* 732.

Townes-Anderson, E., & Raviola, G. 1978. Degeneration and regeneration of autonomic nerve endings in the anterior part of rhesus monkey ciliary muscle. *Journal of Neurocytology, 7,* 583–600.

Uetz, G. W., Kane, T. C., & Stratton, G. E. 1982. Variation in the social grouping tendency of a communal web-building spider. *Science, 217,* 547–9.

Uphouse, L. L., & Bonner, J. 1975. Preliminary evidence for the effects of environmental complexity on hybridization of rat brain RNA to rat unique DNA. *Developmental psychobiology, 8,* 171–8.

Uylings, H. B. M., Kuypers, K., Diamond, M. C., & Veltman, W. A. M. 1978. Effects of differential environments on plasticity of dendrites of cortical pyramidal neurons in adult rats. *Experimental Neurology, 62,* 658–77.

Uylings, H. B. M., Kuypers, K., & Veltman, W. A. M. 1978. Environmental influences in the neocortex in later life. *Progress in Brain Research, 48,* 261–72.

Visintainer, M. A., Volpicelli, J. R., & Seligman, M. E. P. 1982. Tumor rejection in rats after inescapable or escapable shock. *Science, 216,* 437–9.

Volkmar, F. R., & Greenough, W. T. 1972. Rearing complexity affects branching of dendrites in the visual cortex of the rat. *Science, 176,* 1445–7.

Waddington, C. H. 1957. *The strategy of genes.* London: George Allen and Unwin.

Waddington, C. H. 1966. *Principles of development and differentiation.* New York: Macmillan.

Wahler, R. G. 1980. Parent insularity as a determinant of generalization success in family treatment. In S. Salzinger, J. Antrobus, & J. Glick (Eds.), *The ecosystem of the "sick" child: Implications for classification and intervention for disturbed and mentally retarded children.* New York: Academic Press.

Wallen, K. 1982. Influence of female hormonal state on rhesus sexual behavior varies with space for social interaction. *Science, 217,* 375–7.

Walters, L. 1982. Ethical issues in genetic and reproductive engineering. *Abstracts of Papers of the 148th National Meeting of the American Association for the Advancement of Science* (abstract).

Washburn, S. L. (Ed.). 1961. *Social life of early man.* New York: Wenner-Gren Foundation for Anthropological Research.

Washburn, S. L. 1981. Longevity in primates. In J. L. McGaugh, J. G. March, & S. B. Kiesler (Eds.), *Aging: Biology and behavior.* New York: Academic Press.

Washburn, S. L. 1982. Is it sex? *The Sciences, 22,* 2.

Watkins, L. R., & Mayer, D. J. 1982. Organization of endogenous opiate and nonopiate pain control systems. *Science, 216,* 1185–92.

Watson, R. I. 1977. Psychology: A prescriptive science. In J. Brožek & R. B. Evans (Eds.), *R. I. Watson's selected papers on the history of psychology.* Hanover, N.H.: University of New England Press.

Weindruch, R., & Walford, R. L. 1982. Dietary restriction in mice beginning at one year of age: Effect on life-span and spontaneous cancer incidence. *Science, 215,* 1415–18.

Weingartner, H., Gold, P., Ballenger, J. C., Smallberg, S. A., Summers, R., Rubinow, D. R., Post, R. M., & Goodwin, F. K. 1981. Effects of vasopressin on human memory functions. *Science, 211,* 601–3.

Werner, H. 1948. *Comparative psychology of mental development.* New York: International Universities Press.

Werner, H. 1957. The concept of development from a comparative and organismic point of view. In D. B. Harris (Ed.), *The concept of development.* Minneapolis: University of Minnesota Press.

Werner, H., & Kaplan, B. 1956. The developmental approach to cognition: Its relevance to the psychological interpretation of anthropological and enthnolinguistic data. *American Anthropologist, 58,* 866–80.

West, R. W., & Greenough, W. T. 1972. Effect of environmental complexity on cortical synapses of rats: Preliminary results. *Behavioral Biology, 7,* 279–84.

Wetzel, R. 1980. Applications of recombinant DNA technology. *American Scientist, 68,* 664–75.

White, S. H. 1968. The learning–maturation controversy: Hall to Hull. *Merrill–Palmer Quarterly, 14,* 187–96.

Whitehouse, P. J., Price, D. L., Struble, R. G., Clark, A. W., Coyle, J. T., & DeLong, M. R. 1982. Alzheimer's disease and senile dementia: Loss of neurons in the basal forebrain. *Science, 215,* 1237–9.

Willems, E. P. 1973. Behavioral ecology and experimental analysis: Courtship is not enough. In J. R. Nesselroade & H. W. Reese (Eds.), *Life-span developmental psychology: Methodological issues.* New York: Academic Press.

Willer, J. C., Dehen, H., & Cambier, J. 1981. Stress-induced analgesia in humans: Endogenous opioids and naloxone-reversible depression of pain reflexes. *Science, 212,* 689–91.

Williams, G. C. 1966. *Adaptation and natural selection.* Princeton: Princeton University Press.

Willis, S. L. 1982. Concepts from life span developmental psychology: Implications for programming. In M. Okum (Ed.), *New directions for continuing education: Programs for older adults* (No. 14). San Francisco: Jossey-Bass.

Willis, S. L., & Baltes, P. B. 1980. Intelligence in adulthood and aging: Contemporary issues. In L. W. Poon (Ed.), *Aging in the 1980s: Psychological issues.* Washington, D.C.: American Psychological Association.

Wilson, E. O. 1975. *Sociobiology: The new synthesis.* Cambridge: Harvard University Press.

Windle, M., & Lerner, R. M. In press. The role of temperament in dating relationships among young adults. *Merrill–Palmer Quarterly.*

Winick, M. 1980. Nutrition and brain development. *Natural History, 89,* 6–13.

Winick, M., Jaroslow, A., & Winer, E. 1978. Foster placement, malnutrition, and environment. *Growth, 42,* 391–7.

Wise, S. P., & Herbenham, M. 1982. Opiate receptor distribution in the cerebral cortex of the rhesus monkey. *Science, 218,* 387–9.

Wittig, M. A., & Petersen, A. C. (Eds.). 1979. *Sex-related differences in cognitive functioning.* New York: Academic Press.

Wohlwill, J. 1980. Cognitive development in childhood. In O. G. Brim, Jr., & J. Kagan (Eds.), *Constancy and change in human development.* Cambridge: Harvard University Press.

Woolf, N. K., Bixby, J. L., & Capranica, R. R. 1976. Prenatal experience and avian development: Brief auditory stimulation accelerates the hatching of Japanese quail. *Science, 194,* 959–60.

Wright, J. W., & Harding, J. W. 1982. Recovery of olfactory function after bilateral bulbectomy. *Science, 216,* 322–4.

Wurtman, R. J. 1982. Nutrients that modify brain function. *Scientific American, 246,* 50–9.

Yarczower, M., & Hazlett, L. 1977. Evolutionary scales and anagenesis. *Psychological Bulletin, 84,* 1088–97.

Yarczower, M., & Yarczower, B. S. 1979. In defense of anagenesis, grades, and evolutionary scales. *Psychological Bulletin, 86,* 880–4.

Zakon, H., & Capranica, R. R. 1981. Reformation of organized connections in the auditory system after regeneration of the eighth nerve. *Science, 213,* 242–4.

Author index

Aaronson, S. A., 38
Abel, E. L., 114
Abravanel, E., 119
Adams, J. E., 77, 169
Akil, H., 76, 77, 81
Allen, V. L., 1, 5
Anderson, P. W., 4, 5
Anderson, V. E., 33
Anderson, W. F., 19, 20
Andrasik, F., 117
Anisman, H., 118
Appel, M. A., 117
Apfelbaum, M., 71, 72
Archer, S. M., 50
Arendash, G. W., 62
Asanov, N. S., 89
Audibert, A., 79
Averill, A. L., 111
Ayala, F. J., 105

Bakan, D., 30
Baldwin, J. M., ix, 8, 9, 22, 26, 120
Ballenger, J. C., 79
Baltes, M. M., 12, 22, 29, 31, 54–6, 61, 158, 164
Baltes, P. B., 1, 4, 12, 19, 22–31, 54–6, 61, 158, 165
Bandura, A., 23, 55, 112, 160, 161
Barbeau, A., 67, 69
Barbin, G., 63
Barbosa, J. A., 40
Barchas, J. D., 76, 77, 81, 83
Barraclough, C. A., 164
Bartus, R. T., 73
Baskin, D. S., 78
Baskin, R. K., 79
Bateson, P.P.G., 164

Baumrind, D., 135
Bayer, S. A., 52
Beatty, W. W., 76
Beer, B., 60, 73
Belsky, J., 26, 140, 142
Benghezal, A., 79
Bengtson, V. L., 30, 136, 137
Bennett, E. L., 34, 49, 51, 54
Bennett, G. J., 81
Benveniste, R. E., 35
Berg, P., 34, 38, 39, 40, 42, 168
Berkowitz, R., 49, 51
Bernardo, L. S., 59
Bregman, B. S., 59
Berscheid, E., 150
Bertolini, A., 114
Besson, J. M., 76
Birch, H. G., 106, 119, 153, 155
Bishop, P., 80
Bixby, J. L., 114
Black, I. B., 113
Black, J. B., 52
Block, J., 10, 11, 12, 13
Block, J. H., 10, 11, 13, 19, 30
Bock, C. E., 112
Bock, W. J., 99
Bodmer, W. F., 33
Bohn, M. C., 113
Bolles, R. C., 76, 78
Bondareff, W., 59, 61
Bonds, A. B., 50
Bonner, J., 34
Boothe, R. G., 56
Brassard, J. A., 141
Bregman, B. S., 59
Brent, S. B., 1, 10, 29, 126, 138, 139

Bridges, R. S., 81
Brim, O. G., Jr., x, xii, 1, 8, 10, 16, 18, 22–4, 29, 31, 70, 135, 136
Bronfenbrenner, U., 1, 22, 131, 140
Bronson, F. H., 164
Brooks-Gunn, J., 120
Brown, D. D., 40, 168
Brown, M. S., 37
Browne, J., 40, 41
Buech, B. V., 22
Buell, S. J., 58, 59, 164
Bühler, C., 120
Bullough, V. L., 118
Burgess, R. L., 22
Busch, R., 114
Busch-Rossnagel, N., 10, 12, 23, 26, 30, 105, 120, 151, 166, 173

Cairns, R. B., 166, 167
Cambier, J., 83
Campbell, D. T., 27
Campenot, R. B., 47
Capitanio, J. P., 105
Capp, R. H., 68, 69
Capranica, R. R., 47, 114
Carder, B., 77
Carlsmith, J. M., 117
Cavalli-Sfarza, L. L., 33
Chang, F.L.F., 51, 57
Changeaux, J. P., 56
Chen, J., 116
Cherkovich, G. M., 89
Chernick, V., 78
Chess, S., 11, 19, 150, 152–5, 160
Clark, A. W., 58, 59
Clarke, A.D.B., 1, 18, 31, 165

197

Subject index

Acetylcholine, 53, 64, 67, 68
Acetylcholinesterase, 54
ACTH, 76
Active organism, and own perceptual development (*see also* Individuals as producer of own development), 119, 120
Adaptation: definitions of, 99; and effects, 99; and functions, 99
Adaptationist program, 100, 101
Adrenal glands, 63
Age changes, in responsivity to stimuli, 60
Age-graded events, 27
Aging: and biological vulnerability, 55; and decline, 22; and dietary manipulation, 60; mechanisms of, 61; and multidirectional change, 22; and selective optimization, 54, 55
Alleles, 39
Alzheimer's disease, 58, 73
Anagenesis: and complexity, 105; definitions of, 105; and evolutionary grades, 105
Anticipatory socialization, 140
Antigens, 36
Aortic lesions, 118
Aptation, 101; definition of, 100
A/S ratio, 44, 106, 107; and developmental rate, 106; in humans, 44
Assessment: life-span perspective's orientation to, 148; prior to intervention, 148
Association cortex, 44
Atherosclerosis, 37
Attachment, 14, 134, 141
Australopithecines, 90
Axonal plasticity, 60

Behavioral development, Schneirla's definition of, 5
Behavioral interventions, 71, 72
Behavioral plasticity, in the aged years, 54
Beliefs, and intervention, 18–20
Beta-endorphin (*see also* Endogenous opioids),

71; and obesity, 72; and overeating, 71; and passive avoidance, 79
Bidirectional relations, between individual and social context (*see also* Reciprocal relations), 122
Biological development: in adolescence, effects of the social context, 116–18; in infancy, effects of experience, 116
Biological disorders, effects of psychosocial factors, 118
Biological functioning, contextual influences, 113–19
Biological-maturational model of growth, 22
Blood-brain barrier, 68
Bonding: and love, 14; mother–infant, 14
Brain-behavior relations, 1; changes in aging, 59
Brain circuitry: changes, effects of lesion-induced stimulation, 45; flexibility of, 45, 46; long-term changes, 45
Brain development: across life-span, 51, 52; and the use of transplants, 62–4
Brain plasticity (*see also* Synaptic plasticity), 45–57; and aging, 57–62; and critical periods, 54; developmental processes, 55–7; and early experience, 54; and effects of environmental complexity, 54; and role of experience, 45–51; and sensitive periods, 54
Brain structures, effects of dietary restriction (*see also* Synaptic plasticity), 60

Catecholamines, 74
Causality, 1, 15; and brain processes, 2; interactionist interpretation, 2; multilevel view of, 6; and physical and chemical laws, 2
Cerebral cortex, cholinergic innervation of, 59
Cerebral palsy, 146
Change, sources of in probabilistic epigenesis, 27
Child development institutes, 22
Children, as active agents in own development

202